Giving Comfort and Inflicting Pain

by

Irena Madjar

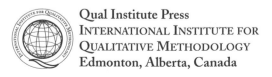

Qual Institute Press
INTERNATIONAL INSTITUTE FOR
QUALITATIVE METHODOLOGY
Edmonton, Alberta, Canada

For information:

 Qual Institute Press
INTERNATIONAL INSTITUTE FOR
QUALITATIVE METHODOLOGY
Sixth Floor
University Extension Centre
8303–112th Street
University of Alberta
Edmonton, Alberta, Canada T6G 2T4
Phone: 1-403-492-9041
Fax: 1-403-492-9040
Email: qualitative.institute@ualberta.ca
Or order books from our website: http://www.ualberta.ca/~iiqm/

Printed in Canada

Canadian Cataloging-in-Publication Data

Madjar, Irena, 1949–
      Giving comfort and inflicting pain
      Includes bibliographical references and indexes.
      ISBN 0-9683044-2-7
      1. Pain. 2. Nursing. I. Title.
      RT87.P35M33 1998   616'.0472   C98-900174-1

Editor: Janice M. Morse
Managing Editor: Don Wells
Graphic Design: Murray Pearson

Contents

Acknowledgements

This book is based on a PhD thesis submitted to Massey University, New Zealand at the end of 1991. Attempts to publish it as a complete monograph have proved frustratingly unsuccessful as various publishing companies decided that a book about clinically inflicted pain lacked sales potential.

In early 1997, a chapter focusing on the phenomenon of clinically inflicted pain and drawing on the material from the thesis was published by Churchill Livingstone in *The Body in Nursing*, edited by Jocalyn Lawler. A further chapter, addressing the problem of the nurses' experience of inflicting pain, will appear in *Phenomenological Inquiry and Nursing Practice*, to be published by Allen and Unwin in 1998. I am delighted, however, that Dr. Janice Morse has encouraged me to submit the manuscript for publication with The Qual Institute Press, so that finally the dissertation will be presented in its entirety. I hope that others will share her sense that despite the passage of time since the original study the book still has something worthwhile to say to nurses and others working with people in pain.

This book is dedicated to the patients and the nurses who have helped me to understand something of what it means to endure pain and to have to inflict it and to Norma Chick, Andrew Trlin, Jo Ann Walton and Janice Morse who have enriched my professional and personal life and in their individual ways ensured that this did not become just another PhD dissertation gathering dust on a library shelf.

Preface

The experience of pain is an intrinsic part of human life, and interest in its alleviation is one of the traditional concerns of nursing. Yet despite the very significant improvements in pain management that have been achieved over recent years, pain remains a challenge to our understanding and resists our attempts to prevent and control it. A particularly urgent challenge is posed by the problem of pain resulting from medically prescribed procedures, which are often carried out by nurses as part of their everyday work. This book is about pain and the infliction of pain, not in the context of abuse or torture, which imply the infliction of bodily pain, but in the context of nursing practice in a hospital setting, that is, in a context more readily associated with caring and relief of pain. Because this aspect of nurses' work is often unacknowledged, there are few rules to guide nurses' practice, and there is little in the way of nursing research that would sensitize nurses to the full implications of those aspects of their work that involve pain infliction.

This book is based on a phenomenological study involving two populations of adult patients and the nurses with direct involvement in their care. One population consisted of people with cancer who experienced a period of intravenous chemotherapy, and the other people were being treated in hospital following burn injuries. These, and other, groups of patients are frequently expected to endure not only pathological pain arising from their disease or injury, but also the pain generated by diagnostic and treatment procedures carried out by nurses or other health care workers. Even when recognized, such pain is often seen as a side-effect—an unintended but inevitable by-product of the legitimate primary tasks of diagnosis and therapy. Thus, it can be argued that some degree of inflicted pain is often both inevitable and necessary if the patient is to be provided with an accurate diagnosis and appropriate treatment. Yet in the lived world of patients' and nurses' experience, deciding what is necessary or unnecessary, avoidable or unavoidable, is fraught with tensions and difficulties.

Unlike pathological pain resulting from disease or injury, clinically inflicted pain has received relatively little attention in the research literature. Such pain can be viewed from at least two perspectives: either from the perspective of the person experiencing the pain or from the perspective of the person who by his or her actions provokes or contributes to the pain experience. Neither perspective has received the research and scholarly attention it deserves from nurses or from other health professionals. This gap in knowledge has important repercussions for both nursing practice and nursing education. In clinical practice, nurses continue to perform procedures that are painful to patients. Yet without an adequate understanding of the nature of inflicted pain and sufficient knowledge about its prevention and management, they are ill-prepared to reduce either the incidence and severity of such pain or their own feelings of stress when having to inflict pain. At the same time, nursing curricula have little, if anything, to say about those aspects of nursing practice that contribute to patients pain, about ethical issues related to pain infliction and pain relief, or about possible implications for nurses as persons who hurt (however unintentionally) those in their care.

In writing this book, my particular concern has been to extend and deepen our understanding of the lived experience of pain, particularly when it is inflicted in the context of medically prescribed treatments. In drawing on the lived experience of the participants, the aims have been to explicate the meaning of inflicted pain as well as its impact, both on patients and on the nurses who are required to perform the potentially painful procedures.

Interest in the study presented in this book was stimulated by an unexpected finding from my earlier research into patients' experience of pain following abdominal surgery (Madjar, 1981). Two-thirds of the 33 participants in that study reported pain originating from sources other than their surgical wound. At least some of this nonwound pain resulted from medical or nursing actions, and patients seemed ill-prepared to cope with it. A literature review at the time identified very few research studies that addressed the issue of procedural or incident pain. The few existing reports tended to relate such pain to specific procedures only or to claim that the difficulties associated with this pain are no different from the difficulties associated with pain resulting from disease or injury. Only one study (Fagerhaugh & Strauss, 1977) identified what was referred to as *inflicted pain* to be a significant clinical problem in many acute hospital settings.

Since 1977, a number of researchers have commented on the incidence and/or intensity of pain related to treatment for premalignant disease (Lowles, Al-Kurdi, & Hare, 1983), cancer therapy (Chapman, Syrjala, & Sargur, 1985; Miser, Dothage, Wesley, & Miser, 1987), and treatment following burn injuries (Choiniere, Melzack, Rondeau, Girard, & Paquin, 1989; Perry & Heidrich, 1982). Such studies provide empirical evidence of the relative frequency with which inflicted and therapy related pain occurs in clinical settings. They also demonstrated a growing concern for a clearer acknowledgement and more effective management of such pain, particularly when research findings consistently show that inflicted pain may not only be overlooked (Lowles et al., 1983), but, even when recognized, is frequently undertreated (Heidrich, Perry, & Amand, 1981; Perry & Heidrich, 1982). The quantitative approaches (often correlational survey or experimental designs) used in almost all research related to clinically inflicted pain may be informative about the incidence and severity of such pain. Regrettably, however, they shed little light on the nature of inflicted pain, on how those experiencing it live with such pain, or, in relation to health professionals, on the problem of having to inflict it.

The implied assumption of much of the existing research is that inflicted pain is no different from other types of acute pain. In challenging this assumption, I wanted to ask patients about their experiences of inflicted pain and how nurses experience the necessity of inflicting that pain. As the researcher, I wanted to consider that inflicted pain, while having qualities in common with other kinds of pain, may also have unique features that make it different. I began the study with the premise that the answers to my questions would come from within the lived experiences of people confronted with situations in which they must either inflict or endure such pain. Consistent with this initial assumption, I used a phenomenological approach to obtain answers to my questions. This approach explores the essential humanness of life experiences as they are for those who live them rather than focusing on abstract and decontextualized definitions devised by the observer. Thus, the focus of the study was on pain and pain infliction as lived experiences rather than as operationally defined variables. The research methods included various forms of dialogue, with which I aimed to uncover the lived experience of clinically inflicted pain in the context in which it occurs.

In the clinical environment of a hospital, inflicted pain has its genesis in the actions of people, such as nurses, normally expected to relieve rather than cause pain. The fact that inflicted pain arises from direct and observable actions of others, rather than from some unobservable pathophysiological processes within the person, raises a number of questions, many of which are still unanswered. For example, what are patients' perceptions of inflicted pain and what meanings does it have for them? How do they live through repeated episodes of such pain? How do nurses, motivated by the desire to care for people and educated to provide comfort and relieve pain and suffering, live through the contrasting experiences of inflicting pain as part of their work? What impact does performing procedures that are frequently painful for the patient have on nurses? How do patients, already suffering from life-threatening illness or severe trauma, manage to endure additional pain associated with their treatment?

In acute hospital settings, inflicted pain is something that many nurses and patients confront daily. Yet there is little evidence in the nursing research literature that the issues and questions surrounding the problem of inflicted pain have been adequately considered. Until the problem is understood more clearly, it will be difficult to change the situation in which both the incidence and the severity of inflicted pain remain a serious and, according to available evidence, poorly managed clinical problem (Kelley, Jarvie, Middlebrook, McNeer, & Drabman, 1984; Siddle, Young, Sledmere, Reading, & Whitehead, 1983). My aim was to deepen the understanding of inflicted pain and to provide a basis for more informed nursing practice.

In this book, the term *clinically inflicted pain* is used to refer to **any pain experienced by patients that is directly related to procedures or tasks performed on them by hospital personnel**. Such pain may be associated with diagnostic, therapeutic or monitoring procedures, particularly those that intrude into the patient's body: for example, in the case of cancer patients, procedures that require the penetration of the skin and other tissues by needles or other instruments in order to obtain samples or to facilitate the administration of diagnostic chemicals or treatment medication. Delayed pain, arising from longer-term effects of therapy such as the use of anticancer drugs (for example, pain associated with mouth ulcers that may follow the administration of certain drugs), is not included in the definition. For patients with burns, the main sources of inflicted pain relate to dressing changes and cleaning and washing burned areas of the body. Additional pain may arise from venepunctures and arterial punctures performed for blood sampling and from physiotherapy.

The purpose of the study discussed in this book was to describe the lived experiences of inflicted pain in the context in which they occur and the meanings that such pain has for those who experience it. A phenomenological approach was used to achieve a deeper understanding of the phenomenon of inflicted pain as it is experienced in the context of medically prescribed treatment. For the patients who took part in this study, that context was the experience of treatment and recovery following burn injuries or the experience of intravenous chemotherapy following a diagnosis of cancer. In the case of nurses, the context was the lived world of their everyday practice within the Burn Care Unit or the Oncology Clinic of a city hospital in New Zealand.

While this study was an exercise in phenomenological research, it did not set out to be a phenomenology of pain. Such an undertaking would have been beyond the scope and resources of this study. Nevertheless, the design and focus of the study are informed by some of the central ideas in phenomenology, in particular, Merleau-Ponty's (1962) concepts of embodiment and intentionality. Focal concerns with the lived experience, in this case of inflicted pain, and with understanding in context follow an established pattern of phenomenological research (Benner, 1984a, 1985; Oiler, 1986). The hermeneutical methods of data analysis and interpretation used to transform the personal experiences of the participants into conceptual categories and essential themes are also informed by a phenomenological research approach (Benner, 1984b; Reinharz, 1983; van Manen, 1990).

The philosophical debate about phenomenology and phenomenological research methods is ongoing. Writers such as Toombs (1987) and van Manen (1990), for example, stress the centrality of "eidetic reduction" and focus on the "general essences" of phenomena. In other words, they seek to understand and describe the general and the universal nature of phenomena, not in relation to a particular context, but in the way the phenomena transcend the context from which they are derived. While such an approach is accepted as valid and needed within nursing scholarship, it was not considered to be appropriate within the scope and aims of the present study. The clinical rather than the philosophical orientation makes the present study more circumscribed in nature. In particular, the study relies on data generated from interviews and observations recorded during a specific 5-month period spent in the clinical field. It relies less on other sources, such as research literature, and makes no use of published fiction, experiential accounts in general literature, or other art forms such as poetry, drama, film or painting, all of which may depict lived human experience and be used in phenomenological research and writing (van Manen, 1990). This study and its findings are presented with the expectation that they will make nurses and others involved in the care of people who are ill or injured more understanding of the patients' experiences of pain. At the same time, it is hoped that nurses and others who may read this book will become more reflective about their own practice, particularly those actions that have the potential to generate or relieve pain.

Chapter 1
The Problem of Pain

Despite advances in the medical and health-related sciences over the last century, pain continues to be seen as an "intriguing puzzle" (Melzack, 1973; Menges, 1984) and a challenge to those entrusted with the responsibility for its relief (Melzack & Wall, 1988). Likening the quest for a clear understanding of the scientific bases of pain to great nineteenth-century explorations, Noordenbos (1987) suggests that there is much about pain that remains unknown and that metaphorically "we are as yet far removed from discovering the sources of the Nile" (p. 150). Nevertheless, in recent years, significant advances have been made in the knowledge of pain aetiology and pain management.

HISTORICAL REVIEW OF THE CONCEPT OF PAIN

From the earliest times, pain has been conceptualized as having both natural and supernatural, or at least mysterious, origins. Pain associated with injury could be seen as related to tissue damage and therefore be regarded as a natural phenomenon. Pain associated with disease, however, was more mystifying. It was more readily thought to result from supernatural forces and as a punishment for sinful or inappropriate behavior.

The concept of pain as retributive punishment for sin dates back to the Assyro-Babylonian and Hebraic civilizations and has been remarkably persistent. The English word pain derives from the Latin word *poena*, which means punishment (Procacci & Maresca, 1984). The idea of pain as a consequence of sin is an integral, even though not always well understood, part of the Christian ethic (Tu, 1980). If, as Lewis (1962) suggests, pain is a human experience that involves a complex interaction of physical, mental, and spiritual processes, then the articulation of such experience entails self-description, which, in turn, reveals attitude, belief, and worldview (Polanyi, 1958). However far the scientific understanding of pain advances, its lived experience and individual interpretation will continue to raise questions about meaning that resist a definitive "scientific" answer (Tu, 1980). While there is no intention to negate or diminish the contributions of modern science to the prevention and relief of pain, the very nature of pain means that it is not a problem ultimately amenable to the solutions of the natural sciences alone.

The concept of pain as a natural phenomenon can be traced to Plato and Aristotle. It is Plato who is credited with the notion of pain as a sensation opposite to that of pleasure. Aristotle, who identified the five basic senses as those of vision, hearing, taste, smell and touch, considered pain to be related to an increased sensitivity in these senses, especially touch. While both Plato and Aristotle are thought to have considered the heart to be the centre of all sensations, it is Aristotle who is credited with the notion of pain as a "passion of the soul" felt in the heart (Procacci, 1980; Procacci & Maresca, 1984). The importance of the central nervous system and the brain as the centre of sensation is found later in the writings of Galen (130-201 AD). The concept of pain remained substantially unchanged until the Renaissance, over a thousand years after Galen. Similarly, the idea of the heart as the center of all sensations persisted well into the eighteenth century (Procacci & Maresca, 1984).

The scientific study of pain, in the modern sense, began in the nineteenth century. By the end of the century, it had contributed to a growing conflict between physiologists and a few early psychologists on the one hand and the majority of philosophers and psychologists on the other. The latter supported the traditional Aristotelian concept of pain and stressed its affective quality, while the former, even though divided among themselves, argued for the idea of pain as a sensory phenomenon (Procacci & Maresca, 1984). It is this division, as well as the rapid advances in the fields of anaesthesia and analgesia, that have contributed significantly to the success of what Caton (1985) calls "the secularization of pain" (p. 493). Others have argued that as a result of the rise of science, with its promise of solutions to human suffering, and the less ready acceptance of pain as spiritually redemptive "Western man" has become increasingly more sensitive to pain and less willing to tolerate it (De Moulin, 1974, p. 540). Whether this is so may be open to debate, but what is evident is that the strongly prevailing views of pain among health professionals are secular and derived from scientific explanations. In other words, pain is considered to be a natural phenomenon, most usefully understood in terms of the underlying physiology and pathology, with some acknowledgment of personal and cultural factors, and generally amenable to medical intervention (Fields, 1987; Luckman & Sorensen, 1980; Wall, 1984). Even though it has been suggested that the confidence in the progress of science and its ability to control nature (including pain) may have diminished over the last half century (Caton, 1985), endeavors to solve the puzzle of pain continue.

RECENT ADVANCES IN THE STUDY OF PAIN

The last 30 years have seen a marked increase in the interest in research on and publications about pain. New analgesic drugs have been synthesized, and new means of drug administration perfected (Barkas & Duafala, 1988; Mather & Phillips, 1986). New technologies are being employed in the areas of nerve stimulation and neurodestructive procedures (Lipton, 1987; Murphy, 1989; Waldman, Feldstein, & Allen, 1987). New types of institutions have been created to alleviate particular kinds of pain, hospices for patients with cancer being the prime example. A rediscovery of the problem of chronic pain has led to the establishment of multidisciplinary teams and pain clinics. The International Association for the Study of Pain was founded in 1973, and in 1975, it began publishing *Pain*, the first scientific journal devoted to the topic. As much as these developments serve to demonstrate the advances made, they also point to the complexity of pain. New questions and problems for research and clinical study continue to be generated, and there is a need for a clearer understanding of pain and more appropriate approaches to its management in clinical settings.

In terms of research and theory development, the definition of *pain* is still being debated (Melzack & Wall, 1988). Part of the definitional problem lies in the fact that it is possible to consider a number of different levels of the pain experience, that is, "one person's pain is another's suffering and still a third's nociception [response of sensory nerves to a noxious stimulus]" (Loeser & Black, 1975, p. 81). The terminology used will vary with the presumed anatomical and/or psychophysiological substratum under discussion. Thus, while it is acknowledged that pain is "real" in the sense that it is felt by a person (Spiro, 1976), the word *pain* is an abstraction, and "in this sense, the word is like *beauty*, having no existence of its own, but having an element common to a variety of specific experiences, and ultimately defined only by the experiencer" (Sternbach, 1974, p. 2).

Definitional problems have been compounded by the debate in the area of conceptual models or frameworks. Unidimensional models, which view pain in neurophysiological stimulus-response terms, have been gradually (but by no means entirely) rejected as inadequate, particularly when leading to the assumption that all aspects of the pain experience (for example, anxiety, medication intake, or activity level) are secondary to the intensity of pain. Recent research has challenged assumptions such as this and has advocated moves away from unidimensional models of pain (Ahles, Blanchard, & Ruckdeschel, 1983; Melzack & Wall, 1988) and from the reductionistic premises of the biomedical model of health (Peele, 1981). While calls for change in clinical practice continue to be made, as in other areas, innovations depend on factors other than the availability of supporting research.

It has been suggested that rather than merely treating pain health professionals should be working toward a goal of positive health since "we are well aware that the control of pain, in and of itself, will not assure the emergence of a sense of well being if pursued in a context devoid of compassion, understanding, meaning, and hope" (Ng, 1980, p. 362). Yet even with greater acceptance of the idea of pain as a complex, multidimensional phenomenon, in clinical practice, pain "continues to be viewed most frequently along an intensity dimension" (Turk & Kerns, 1984, p. 57). Researchers continue to report discrepancies between patients' self-reports of pain and health professionals' inferences of patients' pain (Teske, Daut, & Cleeland, 1983; Walkenstein, 1982). One reason suggested for such discrepancies, which usually result in underestimations of pain and its impact on the patient, is that staff continue to operate on the basis of a "dichotomous, organic versus psychogenic model of pain" (Taylor, Skelton, & Butcher, 1984) rather than on the basis of a more integrated model that recognizes the multifaceted nature of pain.

Research evidence indicates clearly that there is no simple one-to-one relationship between tissue damage or pathological lesion (the supposed nociceptive stimulus) and pain (Merskey, 1980). Even when there is a well-recognized pathology, as in cases of injury, pain is not static but evolves in terms of its location, quality, and intensity, not all of which can be accounted for in terms of the original tissue damage or subsequent inflammatory response (Wall, 1984). Nevertheless, when people report pain, whatever its context may be, they place the experience of pain within the body. In terms of direct experience, pain, unlike fear, anger, or other human experiences, has no referent outside of the body (Scarry, 1985). While a nurse may categorize a patient's pain into a known typology and assess it in relation to the generally expected trajectories (Fagerhaugh & Strauss, 1977), the patient knows the pain directly and is "involved in a radically interior way, feeling the pain *from the inside* and knowing that, although others may have the same disease, it is only *her* body which is affected in this instance" (Gadow, 1980, p. 89).

The International Association for the Study of Pain (IASP) captures some of the qualities discussed so far in a definition adapted from one originally formulated by Merskey in 1973. Although relatively simple, the definition of pain as "an unpleasant sensory and emotional experience associated with actual or potential tissue damage or described in terms of such damage" (IASP, 1979) addresses itself to the complexity of pain by recognizing that pain is not only a sensory but also a psychological experience and therefore more than a neurophysiological event. Second, the definition acknowledges that the experiencing person needs to interpret the experience, whether in terms of its unpleasantness or other qualities. And third, whatever its aetiology or quality, pain is seen as something that is experienced and described as situated within the body. The IASP definition of pain is the one most widely used in research and clinical literature, although even this definition is not without its critics. Melzack and Wall (1988), for example, stress the inadequacy of describing pain as something "unpleasant" since pain is more than merely unpleasant: "What is missing in the word 'unpleasant' is the misery, anguish, desperation and urgency that are part of some pain experiences" (p. 45).

PAIN-RELATED ISSUES IN CLINICAL PRACTICE

While many advances in pain management have occurred in recent years, pain remains a reality for many patients, whether following surgery (Sriwatanakul et al., 1983), during experiences of childbirth (Melzack, 1984), in the course of acute or chronic illness (Bonica, 1980; Donovan, 1982), or in the wake of trauma and ensuing treatment (Perry & Heidrich, 1982). Willingly, or otherwise, patients are frequently required to endure not only the pain of their illness or injuries, but also pain associated with diagnostic and therapeutic procedures performed upon them (Fagerhaugh & Strauss, 1977).

Clinical issues related to pain in patients with cancer

Available evidence suggests that in patients with cancer, where survival may be prolonged with therapy, the incidence of pain remains high, with some 40 percent of patients in the intermediate stages of the disease experiencing pain. In advanced cancer, this figure may be as high as 60 to 80 percent (Ahles et al., 1983). Studies conducted at the Memorial Sloan-Kettering Cancer Center found that 30 percent of the patients required narcotic analgesics to relieve their pain, the incidence increasing to 60 percent in terminally ill patients (Coyle, 1985). While the incidence of pain may be expected to be high in hospitalized patients, Ahles, Ruckdeschel, and Blanchard (1984) report similar findings in a study of 208 consecutive oncology clinic outpatients over a 6-month period. Approximately one third (33.5 percent) of the patients in the study had pain related to neoplastic disease, while a further 6.7 percent had pain stemming from treatment procedures such as surgery. The study also revealed that pain was more prevalent in patients with metastatic disease: for example, over 50 percent of patients with bone metastasis reported pain. By comparison, only 18 percent of patients with lymphoma reported having pain.

It is now generally acknowledged that patients with cancer experience pain as evolving over time, influenced by the changes in the tumor and its progression (Wall, 1984) as well as by the effects of different therapies and, in advanced stages, the complications of cachexia and immobility (Coyle, 1985). Cancer is not one homogeneous disease, and at any one time, a person with cancer may be pain free or experience one or more types of pain. Four main categories of pain syndromes have been identified: 1) *pain related to tumor and its spread,* including invasion of bone, compression or infiltration of nerves, occlusion of blood vessels, obstruction of a hollow viscus as well as infection, inflammation, ulceration and necrosis of pain-sensitive tissues; 2) *pain related to cancer therapy,* including surgery, chemotherapy and radiotherapy; 3) *pain related to debilitation and immobilization,* leading to contractures, bed sores and infections; and 4) *pain unrelated to cancer or its treatment,* such as ongoing arthritis or migraine headaches (Coyle, 1985; McGivney & Crooks, 1984).

It has been suggested that pain is one of the most feared consequences of cancer (Coyle & Foley, 1985), but it can also be a presenting symptom of malignancy, especially in children and young adults (Miser, McCalla, Dothage, Wesley, & Miser, 1987).

In another survey of young patients, Miser and her colleagues (1987) found that with this population cancer pain generally diminishes in the majority of cases following initiation of cancer therapy but is replaced by therapy related pain, in particular, neuropathic pain and pain related to effects of surgery and mucosal inflammation. In fact, the authors state that "the high incidence of oral mucositis found in this survey is a direct reflection of the aggressive chemotherapy and radiation protocols received" by many of the patients (Miser, Dothage, Wesley, & Miser, 1987, p. 81). These findings led Miser and her colleagues to call for improvements in both cancer and therapy related pain management.

In spite of such calls, treatment-related pain in patients with cancer is often overlooked or given a lower priority than pain related to the disease. One explanation, offered in the context of a discussion on pancreatic cancer, is that "pain of iatrogenic origin [caused by medical examination or treatment] is typically overshadowed by the severe and relentless pain of the tumor" (Chapman, 1988, p. 188). Others have suggested that inflicted or therapy induced pain does not bring with it the same feelings of fear and uncertainty as the pain of cancer and that the pain is less problematic since its cause is known, its course predictable, and its duration known to be limited. Nevertheless, these same authors state that as patients with cancer live longer the incidence of treatment-related pain is growing. Treatment-related pain may account for as many as 25 percent of patients referred to a specialist pain clinic (Coyle & Foley, 1985). At the same time, clinical experience with patients who have undergone previous cycles of cancer treatment suggests that these patients "view further treatments with dread, and some refuse to continue potentially life-saving interventions because the personal cost of treatment toxicity is so high" (Chapman et al., 1985, p. 100).

Research also reveals a failure to acknowledge pain associated with cancer therapy. In a study conducted at a cancer institute in Boston, Peteet, Tay, Cohen, and MacIntyre (1986) address the issue of pain characteristics and treatment in 100 consecutive outpatients with cancer. Their finding that 30 percent of the patients had pain is in line with other reported studies (Ahles et al., 1984; Miser et al., 1987), but nevertheless, it gives a limited view of what these patients might have been experiencing in terms of pain. In the Peteet, Tay, Cohen, and MacIntyre study, what was defined as pain was only the pain severe enough to require regular or narcotic medication, and further data collection and analysis were undertaken only in relation to patients whose physicians considered their pain to be due to cancer rather than other factors.

Review articles usually note a general paucity of good research studies on cancer-related pain (Jay, Elliot, & Varni, 1986). They also note a lack of published research in relation to the specific problems of treatment-induced toxicity leading to pain (Chapman et al., 1985; Schreml, 1984).

There is no doubt that chronic pain syndromes such as causalgia or deafferentation pain related to nerve damage during amputations and other types of surgery for cancer can be severe and extremely distressing to the patient and the family who must witness and cope with the patient's misery (Chapman, 1988). Relatively rare complications of particular types of chemotherapy, such as pancreatitis, may be extremely painful and even life-threatening (Schreml, 1984). Long-term effects of treatment, such as aseptic necrosis of bone resulting from prolonged steroid therapy or fibrosis following irradiation, can lead to painful and difficult-to-treat conditions (Chapman, 1988). Such pain can persist even when the patient experiences remission of cancer, or it can make the terminal stages of the illness particularly distressing. In either case, the pain can become the primary focus for both the patient and the caregivers.

Severe intractable pain can indeed overshadow what may be perceived as only the "secondary," "short-lived," "trivial" and "easily managed" pain related to cancer therapy (Schreml, 1984). But to ignore or dismiss some pain because other pain may hurt more or be more difficult to control is neither logical nor helpful to patients who must repeatedly endure it. Personal accounts of patients point to distress experienced not only because of pain, but also because of inadequate analgesia and unnecessary suffering (MacInnes, 1976; Murphy, 1987). Schreml (1984) suggests that when patients have been fully informed, their concerns taken into account, and analgesic measures properly instituted then it may be expected that a potentially painful procedure will be well tolerated. The problem is that even without such support patients expect to endure pain for as long as possible and "medical and nursing staff behavior tends to reinforce this belief" (Bond, 1981, p. 570). Bond's comments are based on research in British hospitals. Research from other English-speaking sources would indicate that this situation is not unique to that country (Fagerhaugh & Strauss, 1977; Madjar, 1981).

Bond (1981) goes on to make the observation that staff expectations of patients' ability to tolerate pain may be altered when they themselves become patients. The tendency of doctors and nurses (when they become patients) to "smuggle" analgesics into the hospital with them may be indicative of their concern that their pain may be undertreated. When relating their own personal experiences of illness or surgery, physicians often comment on the unusual severity of their pain (Donald, 1976), inadequate analgesia after the first 48 hours (Freed, 1975), and their particular sensitivity to pain, which is unlike their patients' usual tolerance for pain and lesser need for analgesia (Chisolm, 1987). The disparity in the assessment of their own and their patients' pain is not the only disparity between subjective and objective perspectives, the former marked by emotional involvement, the latter by scientific detachment. In phenomenological terms, discussed more fully in the next chapter, the disparity also reflects the fundamentally different ways in which we know our own, as opposed to another's, body (Benner & Wrubel, 1989; Gadow, 1989).

Of particular interest to the present study is pain associated with the diagnostic and therapeutic procedures that are an inevitable part of the illness experience for the person with cancer. Surprisingly perhaps, such pain has received even less attention in the literature than other types of therapy related pain. Pain related to invasive procedures is more frequently mentioned in the context of cancer in children (Katz, Kellerman, & Siegel, 1980) and adolescents (Blotcky, 1986) than in adults. The overt distress that children undergoing diagnostic and chemotherapy related procedures display may become distressing to the staff as well as making the performance of procedures more difficult. In such situations, some form of general anaesthetic may be advocated (Forlini, Morin, & Treacy, 1987). While fear and anxiety and even anticipatory vomiting may be a problem in this context, Pinnick (1984), in her study of children undergoing repeated intravenous procedures related to chemotherapy, shows that 88 percent of the children found the procedures stressful, and of these, 75 percent identified the threat of pain as the anticipated harm and the main source of stress. It is not entirely surprising to find that behavioral approaches such as hypnosis, behavioral rehearsal, guided imagery and positive reinforcement have been advocated and used with children undergoing "aversive" procedures (Jay et al., 1986; Katz et al., 1980).

In relation to adults, common procedures such as venepunctures for blood tests and insertion of intravenous needles for chemotherapy receive minimal attention, although more specialized procedures may be discussed. Chapman (1988), for example, suggests that invasive procedures such as percutaneous needle biopsies (insertion of a hollow needle through the skin and other overlying tissues for the purpose of withdrawing a small specimen of tissue for laboratory analysis), needle aspirations (withdrawal of fluid from a cyst or a body cavity through a hollow needle), angiography (a radiological examination of blood vessels following the injection of a radio-opoigue dye), and percutaneous transhepatic cholangiography (a radiological examination of the gall bladder and bile ducts following the injection of a radio-opoigue dye through the abdominal or chest wall and the liver) may be potentially or frankly painful or carry the risk of painful complications. The distress that such procedures cause and the lack of habituation to related pain and anxiety may account for patients' reluctance to have some procedures repeated or their aversion to further therapy (Chapman, 1988).

Clinical issues related to pain in patients with burn trauma

People with burns, the second category of patients involved in the present study, are generally recognized as likely to experience pain, both as the result of injury and as the result of treatment. The context and the suddenness of burn trauma mean that the injured persons, especially young and previously healthy individuals, are often ill-prepared to face the pain of their injuries and the prolonged period of usually painful treatments (David, 1982). Dressing changes are by no means the only sources of pain. Discussing rehabilitation following burns, Johnson and Cain (1985) state that "the adage, *the position of comfort is the position of contracture*, summarizes a basic problem. Patients tend to hold the painful burned area in the least painful position, usually that of least stretch" (p. 48). Physiotherapy designed to reduce and remedy scar contractures may, therefore, be a major source of pain for patients with burns.

Whether in children (Kelley et al., 1984) or adults (Robertson, Cross, & Terry, 1985), recovery from burns involves pain as an almost universal experience. Such pain, according to Bonica (1980), serves no useful function and if not adequately managed can lead to serious physiological and psychological disturbances and complications. Bonica (1980) stated that

> despite its overwhelming clinical importance, no serious research on burn pain has been done and little effort has been spent on devising more effective methods of relieving the pain. This is another serious health care problem in which massive efforts have been made to improve the care of all the other aspects of the disorder but the pain problem has been completely neglected. (p. 7)

One outcome of this neglect is the inconsistency in the management of debridement (removal of foreign substances and injured tissues from burn or other traumatic wounds in order to remove potential sources of infection and to promote healing) and other therapy related pain in different hospitals. Perry and Hiedrich (1982) conducted a survey of 181 physicians, nurses and physiotherapists working in 93 burn units throughout the United States. The respondents were asked to indicate what analgesic (pain relieving) and/or psychotropic (sedative or tranquilizing) medication (if any) they would use in given hypothetical situations involving an adult and a 3-year-old child undergoing a debridement procedure. They were also asked to estimate the patients' pain during the procedure after the recommended pain medication was given. While the majority of respondents estimated that the patients' pain would be moderate, the actual dosages of analgesic medication considered as adequate to achieve this level of pain varied widely. In relation to the child, 17 percent of respondents recommended no opioid analgesia, while 8 percent recommended no medication of any kind. In relation to the adult, two-thirds recommended the use of opioids, but the dosage varied from 30 mg of codeine orally to 35 mg of morphine intramuscularly, "equivalent to a 35-fold difference when the route and the relative potency are considered" (Perry, 1984a, p. 1). Of those who recommended intravenous morphine (18 percent of the respondents), as many were inclined to give 3.5 mg as 14.3 mg. The full range was from 2mg to 25mg. Suggested dosages of intramuscular Meperidine™ (Pethidine™) (for a brief description of all drugs mentioned in text, see Appendix B) ranged from 25mg to 375 mg. In addition to analgesics, 52 percent of the respondents recommended also using psychotropic medication, most frequently Diazepam™. Some considered psychotropic drugs, without the addition of any analgesics, adequate. The reasons for such inconsistencies in approach are complex and poorly understood. Perry and Heidrich (1982) suggest that deficiencies in knowledge about pain and the pharmacology of analgesic and psychotropic medication may provide a partial explanation.

Undertreatment of pain

Available research evidence supports Bonica's (1980) claim that pain may be inadequately managed for many patients in acute care settings receiving otherwise sophisticated professional care. Inadequate management may take many forms: for example, pain may be ignored when the therapeutic intervention contributing to it becomes common place (Coates, 1986) or overlooked when new technology is employed without the impact of its use on the patient being assessed (Lowles et al., 1983). Acute pain may also be undertreated when inadequate knowledge, erroneous assumptions and unfounded fears guide clinical practice (Beyer, De Good, Ashley, & Russell, 1983; Mather & Mackie, 1983; Morgan, 1986). Furthermore, while the problems of crosscultural communication are readily recognized, although not always adequately addressed (Madjar, 1985), problems of communication can also arise between patients and caregivers (and among caregivers), even when they belong to the same cultural group. The outcome, once again, is underestimation and undertreatment of pain (Teske et al., 1983).

A further reason for inadequate treatment of pain is the low priority given to the relief of pain in some clinical settings. This is particularly likely in situations where pain serves a useful diagnostic function and its elimination may deprive staff of information deemed to be sufficiently important to warrant withholding pain relief measures: for example, in patients with severe headache following cerebral hemorrhage (Adelman, 1984). Similar principles of priority setting may account for the failure to consider pain assessment and relief in the context of care for burned patients in the first few days of treatment. Robertson and her colleagues (1985), for example, acknowledge that for the patient with burn trauma pain can be all consuming, exhausting and punitive. Nevertheless, their advice is that in the early stages pain-relieving medication should not be given as it can interfere with later attempts to evaluate mental status (Robertson et al., 1985).

When discussing the early nursing care of burned patients, Wooldridge-King (1982) specifies the need to stop the burning process, evaluate the patency of the airway, treat cardiovascular instability, assess for other injuries, assess the burn wound, and institute infection control to prevent further wound contamination. Her only statement about pain is a reminder that "patients with full-thickness injuries experience little or no pain as their sensory nerve endings have been destroyed" (Wooldridge-King, 1982, p. 360). Other relevant points, for example, that patients may also have first- and second-degree burns and even full-thickness burns have wound margins where the depth of the burn may be variable, seem to have been completely overlooked. The only reference to pain relief is that "small intravenous doses of morphine sulphate are usually effective in controlling pain" (Wooldridge-King, 1982, p. 360). It should be noted that research evidence challenges the two points on pain made by Wooldridge-King. For example, a study of 52 randomly selected adult patients in a burn care unit showed that "patients with third-degree burns do have severe pain during procedures" and that procedural pain was inadequately controlled by a mean dose equivalent to 8.9 mg of morphine sulphate administered prior to each procedure (Perry, Heidrich, & Ramos, 1981, p. 324). Clinical evidence from nurses working in a pediatric burn care unit also confirms that "children with third-degree burns do experience severe pain, particularly during procedures" (Atchison, Guercio, & Monaco, 1986, p. 401).

An even more disturbing example of the failure to consider pain and its alleviation in the context of burn trauma is a 339 page textbook on the treatment of burns (Cason, 1981). In its 13 chapters, the author, a physician, discusses prevention, first aid, treatments for various types of burns, likely problems and complications, and rehabilitation. The need for pain relief receives no mention at all, while at the same time, the author gives specific warnings against the administration of narcotics either for restlessness (p. 32) or for "alleged" pain (p. 221).

Given the above examples, it is difficult to avoid the conclusion that in some clinical settings pain and its relief are either ignored, given a very low priority, or taken for granted. Whatever the case may be in a specific situation, patients with burns are likely to experience considerable pain related to their injuries and treatment procedures. Such pain is also likely to be inadequately managed, which can result in increased suffering for the patient. This general conclusion is supported by Fagerhaugh and Strauss (1977), who also note a lack of attention to pain management in the medical literature on the care of patients with burns. These authors suggest that such oversight is understandable (and by implication, acceptable) when it is recognized that even though surrounded by pain the staff in burns units have other, more pressing priorities and are limited in their capacity to relieve patients' pain.

Perry (1984b) suggests that the situation related to the undertreatment of pain may be rather more complex. Reflecting on his attempts to make staff more aware of patients' pain, and using the framework of psychoanalytic theory, he concludes that the phenomenon of undermedication cannot be adequately explained by such factors as staff insensitivity, inadequate knowledge about drugs, or fears of iatrogenic addiction. He goes on to suggest that pain fulfills a deep seated need in patients and staff, reassuring both that despite the damage to the surface of the body the patient's essential self is still there and is alive. The undermedication for pain, and even pain infliction, may provide such reassurance and serve the purpose of preserving the self-object differentiation, declaring who is sick and who is well, since "there is nothing like pain to confirm that the one who is hurting is the one who is ill" (Perry, 1984b, p. 312). Perry offers his observations as professional opinion rather than as conclusions of systematic research. Such professional opinion is difficult to refute, but it does suggest that the phenomenon of pain relief as nursing work is far from fully or clearly understood.

INFLICTED PAIN IN CLINICAL PRACTICE

It is generally accepted that the majority of health personnel working with the ill and injured believe they contribute to the patients' welfare and reduce rather than add to their suffering. In terms of pain management, nurses and physicians feel they are directly involved with the relief of existing pain and the prevention of further pain. It is something of a paradox, therefore, that it is these health professionals who are also, and not infrequently, responsible for inflicting pain in the process of their work on patients.

The scarcity of research on treatment related pain has already been discussed. The dearth of literature dealing with inflicted pain is even more pronounced, and the term itself is seldom used in clinical or research reports. Even in papers that address the issue of treatment-related pain, the emphasis is on the longer-term, drug- or radiation-induced problems, while the immediate impact of procedures performed by health personnel is barely mentioned (Chapman et al., 1985; Coyle & Foley, 1985). With continual introductions of new and sophisticated technology, patients are subjected to more invasive procedures (Abu-Saad, 1984), yet such procedures are not necessarily evaluated for their impact on the patient prior to their general use in clinical practice.

A group of British authors (Siddle et al., 1983), for example, report a study of 58 patients undergoing "Vabra suction curettage," a technique involving the insertion of an instrument through the uterine cervix and the use of suction to obtain tissue samples from the uterine lining. The procedure is used for pretreatment assessment or routine monitoring. The study found that 88 percent of the women experienced pain during the procedure, the level of pain being unrelated to preprocedure anxiety scores. (An earlier study by the same team showed that all 30 women undergoing the procedure experienced pain; 23 percent reporting the pain as severe or very severe, despite a detailed description of the procedure beforehand and the use of distraction during the procedure.) The controlled trial with the 58 women showed that Naproxen Sodium™ did not reduce the severity of pain associated with the procedure (Siddle et al., 1983). Despite the high incidence of pain associated with the procedure, the authors report that the standard practice in Great Britain is to perform the procedure without any form of analgesia or anaesthesia.

Another group of British gynecologists report a retrospective study of 239 women who had undergone carbon dioxide laser treatment for premalignant disease of the uterine cervix. The procedure takes between 5 and 30 minutes (average 15 to 20) and was performed without analgesia or anaesthesia in all women included in the study. Over a period of several years, the operating gynecologist had become aware "that for some women treatment, although tolerated, was a considerable trial" (Lowles et al., 1983, p. 1158). Despite the fact that the questionnaire focused solely upon "significant pain," only 15 percent of the women reported having no pain, while 42 percent reported their pain to have been moderate or severe. Over 30 percent continued to experience pain during the 24 hours after treatment, and 25 percent sought relief by resorting to analgesic medication. A quarter of the group felt the procedure should be done under some form of anaesthetic. Even so, the authors conclude that "the pain is short-lived and ends when treatment stops, and for many it is more acceptable than the inconvenience of a general anaesthetic" (p. 1159). However, they went on to concede that general anaesthesia should be offered more readily to some women and other forms of analgesia investigated (p. 1159).

At other times, research studies of patients' responses to potentially painful procedures adopt definitions and study designs that avoid even the mention of the word pain. In a study of 115 children with cancer undergoing bone marrow aspirations (BMA), Katz et al. (1980) focused on "behavioral distress" prior to, during, and immediately following the procedure.

The researchers conclude that 97 percent of the children "exhibited behavioral anxiety during the actual procedure...confirming the notion that BMA procedures are stressful for virtually all these children with cancer" (Katz et al., 1980, p. 361). The study also produced strong evidence that children do not become habituated to the procedure, challenging the views of some clinicians who believe that as they are repeated bone marrow aspirations become easier for children to tolerate. Noting that children's scores on the behavioral rating scale showed no consistent changes while the nurses' ratings of children's anxiety did tend to drop, the authors (Katz et al., 1980) conclude that

> this marked discrepancy between the child's actual behavior and the observations of the caregiver may be due to the desire of a nurse or doctor inflicting pain and discomfort to view patients as getting used to the procedure. (p. 364)

The point of particular interest here is not only the researchers' conclusion about the discrepancies between actual behaviors and the caregivers' inferences about the children's experience, but also that the just quoted statement appears in the last paragraph of their report, and this is the first and *only* indication given in the report that the bone marrow aspiration is, in fact, painful for the child.

Given nursing's concern with the care and comfort of the ill and the injured, one might expect that the nursing literature would give greater prominence to the effects of painful procedures on patients. Frequently, however, this is not the case. A comprehensive review of the experience of bone marrow transplantation from a nursing perspective (Hutchinson & King, 1983), for example, outlines the history, methods, and results of bone marrow transplantation, and it describes procedures such as the intravenous and intrathecal (within the membranes of the spinal cord, usually the subarachnoid space) administration of drugs, bone marrow aspirations, and likely complications recognized as painful. Consideration of pain management is limited to the statement that parenteral (injected) opioids may be given, while there is not even a mention of how the patient may be prepared for or assisted through the many pain-inducing episodes of recovery, which even without complications lasts many months.

A similar failure to consider pain and its impact on the patient is evident in a review article by Bayley (1990) entitled "Wound healing in the patient with burns." The nurse-author makes no mention of pain, even while stressing the technical aspects of wound care and advocating "gentle handling and careful [dressing] removal techniques" to "prevent disruption of epithelial cells during dressing change" (Bayley, 1990, p. 209).

Despite the inadequate attention to the problem of inflicted pain in the medical and nursing literature, it is clear that patients in many different settings endure such pain (Fagerhaugh & Strauss, 1977; Krant, 1980). They do so even when the experience becomes overwhelming for the observers. For example, in their study of pain behavior in children undergoing debridement procedures following burns, Kelley et al. (1984) report that "although all involved in this research have had much previous exposure to children and adults suffering from illness and trauma, on several occasions observers became faint" (p. 157). The point not acknowledged by the authors is that the observers are free to leave a situation that they find distressing, but the patients are not. Patients with burns, and those being treated for cancer, are seldom free to leave a situation regarded by their caregivers as necessary. Unless a person refuses all treatment, whether in a burns unit or oncology setting, he or she is going to experience some inflicted pain as an inevitable part of treatment.

A study of 42 adult patients admitted to two burn centers in Montreal highlights the problem of inflicted pain (Choiniere et al., 1989). Even though 76 percent of the patients received an average dose of 6.5 mg of morphine intramuscularly prior to treatment procedures, over half reported intense pain during procedures: 16 percent rating their pain "unbearable." The results showed that there was no significant correlation between pain scores and burn size, duration of hospitalization, or patient's age, educational level, or socioeconomic status. Furthermore, while patients who scored higher on anxiety and depression measures reported more background pain, during treatment, there was no significant correlation between anxiety or depression scores and the reported intensity of inflicted pain. The study concludes that "the most intense pain in burned patients does not relate as much to the burn injury itself as to the trauma caused by the therapeutic procedures [and] that standard and inflexible doses of narcotics are quite likely to be inadequate in burned patients" (Choiniere et al., 1989, p. 1537), which confirms that in clinical situations inflicted pain remains a problem that is still inadequately managed. Greater relief of such pain could be achieved through the more frequent use of continuous intravenous infusion of narcotics, especially in the form of patient-controlled analgesia, the use of inhalation analgesics and subanaesthetic doses of Ketamine™, and the use of techniques such as hypnosis and stress reduction (Marvin & Heimbach, 1985). However, research evidence and clinical observation suggest that such relief measures are still not widely accepted. Underlying this lack of acceptance may well be a poor understanding of the nature of inflicted pain and its impact on the patients.

The pioneering work of Fagerhaugh and Strauss (1977), who reported on the phenomenon of inflicted pain within a broader study of pain in hospitalized patients, remains the most comprehensive statement on the nature of the interactive processes involved in the generation and endurance of clinically inflicted pain. Their discussion is focused on the experience of patients in a specialized burn care unit. Given its relevance to the study in this book, both in terms of the subject matter and the research method used, Fagerhaugh and Strauss' work is reviewed here in some detail.

Fagerhaugh and Strauss (1977) used a grounded theory approach, extensive periods of participant observation, and patient and staff interviews. They suggest that inflicted pain is very common and that a considerable proportion of nurses' work with or around patients includes the inflicting of pain.

For the staff, inflicted pain was almost always a *secondary consideration* since it occurred mainly as a by-product of the more central diagnostic, monitoring, therapeutic, or even comfort-giving work. The legitimate nature of the primary medical or nursing work, accepted by both staff and patients, in turn gave legitimacy to the infliction of pain, which in any other situation might be viewed as an assault on the person. Such a view justifies the infliction of pain because it is necessary in order to accomplish the primary tasks or goals of patient care, but it also results in the prevention and relief of inflicted pain being given a lower priority. Fagerhaugh and Strauss accepted the legitimacy and inevitability of inflicted pain, although they did question whether all such pain was necessary. It is worth noting that while they did not document the details of pain management strategies employed with the burn patients they accepted staff's concerns about the sedative and addictive properties of opioid medication as apparently reasonable grounds for both the insufficient relief of inflicted pain and the lower priority given to it. New developments in the areas of analgesic medication and drug delivery systems over the last two decades require that such views be questioned and revised if inflicted pain is to be managed more effectively.

Fagerhaugh and Strauss also found that when the necessity to inflict pain became a part of the patient-staff interaction an *implicit contract* developed between the two parties. They conclude, therefore, that inflicted pain is best understood as a complex interactive process. Unless coercion is used, the contract implies that the patient will cooperate with the procedure and control pain expression at a level acceptable to the staff. The patient is obliged to endure inflicted pain for as long as possible and keep pain expression within proper bounds. For example, a patient may grunt or moan but not scream loudly or move in a way that interferes with the staff's performance of the task. In the case of an incompetent or negligent performance on the part of a particular staff member, the patient may complain but only if the above obligations have been met; otherwise, the patient runs the risk of being scolded or labeled as uncooperative and difficult. For the staff, the main task was to get the procedure done, however much pain or discomfort that created. They usually explained the necessity of the procedure and the inevitability of concomitant pain, but they also persuaded and encouraged or shamed, chided, scolded, or even threatened patients (particularly children) in order to get the job done.

Whatever other impact they may have observed, according to the authors, "Most of the staff's tactics are devoted to getting the patient to endure and to keep expression from interfering too much" (Fagerhaugh & Strauss, 1977, p. 91). In this use of tactics and countertactics, patients used delay, information or reassurance seeking, attempted to control the situation by issuing instructions to the staff, and sometimes threatened to discontinue treatment if the procedures were too painful. While nurses new to such work had difficulties both in inflicting pain and in handling its expression, the more experienced nurses tended to be better able to tolerate patients' behavior, providing it did not interfere with the performance of the task at hand.

Fagerhaugh and Strauss found that the handling of the inflicted pain by the patients and staff was influenced by a number of factors. The pain itself, in terms of its predictability, intensity, duration and frequency of repetition, was important. Just as important were factors related to treatment procedures that resulted in pain, especially when such procedures were frequent or there were difficulties in their performance. Nurses' skills, concerns for particular patients, presence of fatigue, pressures of other work, and the quality of relationships with patients and other staff were yet another set of factors to be considered. And finally, patients' state of health, fatigue, and previous experiences with particular staff and particular procedures also needed to be taken into account when trying to understand patients' and nurses' experiences of inflicted pain. The findings point to the complexity of inflicted pain, which goes beyond incidence rates and intensity scores.

The findings of Fagerhaugh and Strauss from a burn care unit also suggest that patients admitted into such a setting are socialized by staff and fellow patients to accept their situation. Patients are expected to accept the pain and the extent to which it may or may not be relieved and to adopt an acceptable style and level of pain expression so that the sentimental order of the ward is not disrupted. Sentimental order refers to "the intangible but very real patterning of mood and sentiment that characteristically exists on each ward" (Fagerhaugh & Strauss, 1977, p. 290), and it includes staff morale, quality of informal relationships among staff, and the degree to which formal rules are applied, particularly in dealing with patients and their families.

These researchers found that while the patients with burns described severe and sometimes almost intolerable pain their behavior expressed little of the extent of their suffering. Initially, the situation seemed baffling: "The relative absence of pain expression on this ward was not only striking, but somewhat unreal" (Fagerhaugh & Strauss, 1977, p. 101). This observation became understandable when the research revealed that on this ward "the salient pain tasks, both for patients and staff, are the *enduring of pain* and the *controlling of pain expression*" (p. 101). A patient who lacked self-control and cried or screamed freely when in pain could have a demoralizing impact on both staff and other patients. Thus, the pressure to conform came from both staff and other patients, requiring that all behave within acceptable limits of pain expression. One is led to the conclusion that if the pain were to be managed more effectively then patients would have less pain to endure and staff would need to put less energy into controlling pain expression.

The study also revealed that nurses tended to focus on the technical aspects of care and the immediate treatment situations rather than on the long-term outcomes of treatment or the psychosocial needs of patients. Technical competence was accorded high priority and prestige, while pain management received minimal attention. Staff tended to assess the pain as less severe than the patients' own assessments of it and attributed most of the patients' overt distress to anxiety rather than pain. Even so, staff discouraged patients' expressions of anxiety about their likely futures, and patients accepted that expressions of anxiety might have a negative impact on other patients. The more experienced nurses tended to give smaller doses of medication prior to painful procedures and were less concerned about inflicting pain than the less experienced nurses.

The extent to which the implicit contract between staff and patients ensured behavioral conformity and maintained the usual sentimental order of the ward became apparent when one patient refused to conform to others' expectations. A patient described by the researchers as "articulate and medically sophisticated" (Fagerhaugh & Strauss, 1977, p., 110), who contested staff's treatment and pain management approaches, affected not only staff, but also other patients. Encouraged by his example, other patients expressed their concerns and displeasure about care, upsetting the sentimental order of the ward and frustrating attempts by staff to elicit usual levels of cooperation from the patients.

The researchers conclude that without changes the situation in which there is "too much unnecessarily inflicted pain" will persist, and "the cycles of resentment and distrust generated by even quite necessary pain" will continue (Fagerhaugh & Strauss, 1977, p. 86). Their proposed solutions are largely organizational: "more *communication* to and from patients, genuine *staff focus on pain work* other than the obvious inflicted pain and its limited relief, and similar administrative *accountability* for pain management that is demanded for medical and procedural matters" (p. 112).

NURSING PRACTICE AND PAIN MANAGEMENT

Knowledge about pain and the means to alleviate it alone does not provide either nursing or medicine with a sufficient basis for adequate pain management. Both nursing and medicine are not only scientific and practice disciplines, they are also moral enterprises (Benner & Wrubel, 1989; Jonsen, 1978). Both accept the Hippocratic injunction "to help, or, at least, to do no harm" (MacKinnon, 1988, p. 314). While not every instance of inflicted pain is perceived or experienced as harmful, the moral questions need to be asked: For example, how much inflicted pain can be justified, even if the action producing the pain is done entirely for the benefit of the patient? What are the limits of endurance required of patients in particular clinical situations, what should be the limits, and who should decide on the expected limits for individual patients? Such questions are raised in bioethical discussions (Copp, 1985; Edwards, 1984; Gadow, 1986), but they are seldom debated either in the scientific literature on pain management or in clinical settings. One result of this paucity of ethical debate is that in relation to pain management patients' autonomy is often subjugated to professional paternalism. Patients may be given little latitude over decisions on pain management, and their individual capacity and willingness to endure pain may receive minimal attention (Engelhardt, 1980). In the meantime, as the preceding discussion has shown, patients continue to experience significant pain, including inflicted and unnecessary pain.

It might be tempting to conclude that the high incidence of inflicted pain in hospital settings is the result of insensitive and uncaring staff. The research does not support such a simplistic conclusion. After 8 years of working in a specialist burn care unit and ongoing research in the field, Perry (1984b) found no evidence that undermedication for pain resulted from staff wishing patients to experience pain. On the contrary, he cites a study conducted in the unit that showed a high degree of stress among nurses who were frequently upset by the need to perform painful procedures on patients. Despite this, the nurses continued to perform the procedures and to provide analgesic medication in doses inadequate for pain relief. In another article, Perry (1984c) concludes that "an interesting paradox is the staff's genuine interest in relieving burn pain and yet their tendency to administer analgesics at ineffective dosages" (p. 194).

Perry's (1984b) professional opinion that the presence of pain fulfills a deep-seated need in patients and staff for confirmation of aliveness and differentiation between the healthy and the ill has already been mentioned. A noted medical ethicist offers a different interpretation when he suggests that "when good persons possess great powers and wield them on behalf of others, they sometimes fail to recognize the harm done as they ply their beneficent craft" (Jonsen, 1978, p. 832). Common human frailties of fatigue, of being able to carry only so much responsibility, of timidity or fear that stops us from questioning orders or advocating on behalf of the powerless may also lead to situations in which nurses not only fail to relieve another's pain, but become part of its cause (Anton, 1984; Dind, 1985).

Nursing in particular espouses values that stress caring (Benner & Wrubel, 1989; New Zealand Nurses Association, 1984) and the exercise of its art with due consideration for the safety and welfare of persons in its care (Styles, 1982). Caring within nursing, however, may involve priorities that do not place high value on pain prevention and relief. Thus, it is possible for patients and nurses to develop different perspectives of the patient's experience and different priorities and expectations in relation to nursing actions.

One of the prime expectations that patients have in relation to nursing activities is that of comfort and relief of discomfort (White, 1972). More recent studies of caring within nursing practice report that hospitalized patients perceive "relief of pain and assistance with pain management" as one of the major indicators of caring (Brown, 1986). A study of cancer patients identified skilled performance of physical procedures such as intramuscular injections and venepunctures as one of the five most important nurse caring behaviors (Mayer, 1986). A review of several studies showed that patients' family members identified "nurses' efforts to make the patient comfortable" and "teaching the family how to keep their relative physically comfortable" as two of the ten most helpful nurse caring behaviors (Mayer, 1986, p. 63). When asked for examples of noncaring nursing actions, patients have provided descriptions of experiences that focus on "insensitivity and treating the patient as an object" and "being rough in their physical handling of the patient and belittling in their attitudes" (Riemen, 1986b).

Some studies report a significant correlation between nurses' and patients' perceptions of caring, particularly in relation to factors such as listening to the patient, anticipating patients' needs, and being available to the patient (Mayer, 1986). However, while patients and family members also emphasize relief of symptoms such as pain and discomfort and recognize the difference between skilled and unskilled performance of potentially painful tasks such as intramuscular and intravenous injections, nurses have not identified these as particularly significant indicators of caring (Mayer, 1986; Wolf, 1986). One finds considerable ambivalence in nursing literature about the significance of pain in nurses' work and the extent to which nursing is responsible for the management and relief of patients' pain. Fagerhaugh and Strauss (1977) posit that one of the key reasons for inadequate pain management in hospitalized patients is the lack of staff accountability for other than the technical aspects of their work. Nurses may perform painful procedures, they may administer some form of analgesic medication, and they may be called to task if there is evidence of incompetence or negligence in their technical performance. Yet they do not report to any one nor are they held accountable for the quality of the patients' experience during the procedure or the amount of pain they cause the patient. The situation may vary in different clinical settings.

In areas such as specialized oncology nursing, there is considerable emphasis on the management of the patient's symptoms, including pain (Hauck, 1986; Welch-McCaffrey, 1986). Elsewhere, and especially perhaps in the early stages of trauma care and in critical care units, pain may receive low priority and inadequate attention (Bryan-Brown, 1986; Robertson et al., 1985; Solem, 1987). In some circumstances, nurses may give priority to reinforcing bravery in the face of pain and controlling pain expression rather than to pain prevention or relief (Bond, 1981; Fagerhaugh & Strauss, 1977).

Historically, pain has shifted from being one of the central concerns of nursing to a less well-defined place within the statements on the nature and scope of nursing. The commitment to the relief of pain and suffering is evident in much of the classical nursing literature. Nightingale (1970), in a book first published in 1859, for example, states that it is the duty of the nurse to supply whatever help is needed by a suffering person; Orlando (1961) stresses the assurance of physical and mental comfort as one of the principal tasks of nursing; and Travelbee (1971) states that the purpose of nursing is to help individuals or groups "prevent or cope with the experience of illness or suffering" (p. 16). Such literature also focuses on the person who is ill, "the patient," literally, the one who endures suffering or pain (Caton, 1985). By contrast, the more recent nursing literature deliberately chooses to refer to "clients" (Newman, 1986) or "health care consumers" or even more generally to "persons" (Gottlieb & Rowat, 1987). While there are good reasons for this change in terminology, there is no doubt that the change exemplifies a move away from concerns with illness and suffering and the related focus on relief of pain and discomfort toward a much broader perspective, within which pain is less central.

The move to establish nursing as an independent discipline different from medicine has produced new perspectives on the work of nursing and the relationship with those nursed. The more recent emphasis in statements on nursing has been on health as a process of actualization of human potential and on the nursing's concern with the maintenance and enhancement of wellness (Newman, 1986; Parse, 1987). While emphasizing caring and human interaction, such conceptualizations of nursing give prominence to ideas of "expanding consciousness" (Newman, 1986) and principles of "cocreating reality and cotranscending life situations" (Parse, 1987). These conceptualizations of nursing give less specific prominence to nursing's responsibility for the identification and relief of human pain and suffering in the context of trauma, illness and medical treatment.

A significant exception to this trend is provided by Benner (1984a) and Benner and Wrubel (1989), who argue for the "primacy of caring" in nursing but at the same time see pain and suffering as a frequent concomitant of illness and their relief as one of the key domains of nursing practice. Benner and Wrubel (1989) present caring as "always specific and relational" (p. 3) and as having persons, experiences and events matter to people. To the nurse, then, the primacy of caring implies an ongoing concern with the patient as a person whose specific experiences, feelings and desires matter and are points of connection between the patient and the nurse. Because a patient's experience matters to the nurse, it "sets up the possibility for giving help and receiving help" (Benner & Wrubel, 1989, p. 4). Such a formulation of nursing offers the possibility for more effective communication between patients and nurses and interventions that are more responsive to the patient's individual experience, including the experience of pain. In relation to the problem of inflicted pain, Benner and Wrubel's formulation of nursing offers a further possibility for acknowledging that the nurse's experience of inflicting pain also matters and does not need to be suppressed as seems often to be the case. Stressing the primacy of caring in nursing and positing caring as a moral art provide a framework for nursing practice within which knowledge, personal experience and moral concerns can all be given full attention in determining nursing actions, including those directed at pain management.

Chapter 2
The Case for Phenomenology in the Study of Human Embodiment and Pain

Much of present day research on pain is conducted within the paradigm of traditional science, with its emphasis on testing hypotheses derived from existing theories and on quantification and data analysis through statistical manipulation (*Pain*, 1975–1997). Such research is heavily reliant on laboratory studies and the use of animal models, and it focuses primarily on mechanisms of nociception and the intensity dimension of pain. Even in clinical research, pain, which is among the most subjective and private of human experiences, is frequently operationalized and reduced to observable behaviors or measurable indicators that facilitate the particular research but fail to capture the complexity and richness of the human experience of pain.

Such research is both useful and necessary, yet by defining the phenomenon of pain as a series of biophysiological or behavioral events, it can answer only a limited range of questions about it. Traditional scientific research has said little about pain as a lived human experience in the context of trauma, illness and therapy. By its emphasis on objectification and quantification of pain, it has tended to offer a particular perspective on what it is to be a person and the nature of human embodiment. However, as Benner and Wrubel (1989) point out, the mechanistic model of the person underlying much of the biological and social science study of human activity is often taken for granted to such an extent that its assumptions are seldom made explicit and the implications of its adoption rarely considered.

The mechanistic model, stemming from the Cartesian notion of mind-body dualism, assumes a physical body extrinsic to the essential self, and one that is driven by mechanical causes and open to mathematical analysis (Leder, 1984). Personal meanings are seen as both idiosyncratic and inaccessible in any direct way to another person and, therefore, as largely out of the domain of scientific study or of interest to scientists only when generalizable to categories or groups of people (Benner & Wrubel, 1989). The prevailing view in Western medicine, according to some critics, is that of the patient's body as an object and of the patient as the mere possessor of the body, who hands it over to those with the necessary knowledge to work on it and repair it (Bologh, 1981).

It is evident from much of the research literature that pain continues to be regarded as a phenomenon that can and should be objectified. Klein and Charlton (1980), for example, undertook a study of pain in critically burned patients that they deliberately limited to direct observations of patients' unsolicited verbal and nonverbal behaviors during treatment procedures in order to "avoid patient's rationalizations and other distortions which are often produced with self-report measures" (p. 28). Observed behaviors were classified into two main categories of "complaint" (which included a subcategory of "complaint of pain") and "well-being." All recorded behaviors were given "equal weight," tallied and then analyzed. The results indicated that on the average patients demonstrated more "well-being" than "complaint" behaviors. Even though the authors acknowledged that patients experienced "prolonged, severe pain," the implication was that the high rate of "wellness" behaviors indicated that the procedures were not as painful as studies that have utilized patients' self-reports of pain might indicate. Klein and Charlton (1980) also suggest that with appropriate behavioral reinforcement the rate of "wellness" behaviors may be further increased and the rate of "complaint" behaviors decreased (pp. 28–30). The assumptions and practical consequences of such an approach to pain are in line with a view of the person as an object, focusing on that which is open to the observer's scrutiny and negating the significance of individual patient's perceptions, meanings and experiences. Among its other shortcomings, such a view gives preeminence to observable data and fails to recognize that physical events associated with reports of pain "only serve to make a report of pain more acceptable to us [the observers]. They do not prove its occurrence" (Merskey, 1982, p. 11).

Another way in which research studies objectify pain is to reduce it to a single quantifiable measure that can then be correlated with similarly quantifiable measures such as patients' age, amount of tissue damage, anxiety scores, or staff assessments of patients' pain (Perry, Cella, Falkenberg, Heidrich, & Goodwin, 1987; Van der Does, 1989). Correlational studies try to explain pain and its severity or persistence on the basis of apparent links with a range of isolated physiological and psychosocial variables. The results of such research have failed to demonstrate any consistent relationship between pain intensity during painful procedures and such variables as: patients' psychiatric history or history of drinking problems (Klein & Charlton, 1980); age, ethnicity, education, occupation, extent and location of burns, or length of hospitalization (Perry et al., 1981); or anxiety and depression scores, socioeconomic status, severity of initial injury, or time since the injury (Choiniere et al., 1989). Studies using unidimensional measures of pain to compare patients' and nurses' assessment of patients' pain have produced similarly equivocal results (Iafrati, 1986; Van der Does, 1989; Walkenstein, 1982). Despite inconclusive findings that offer few answers to those who have to deal with pain in clinical situations, this type of research continues to be reported. The appropriateness of research design and methods used in such studies is seldom questioned by their authors.

There have been those who have called for a change of perspective in the study of pain. Merskey (1982), for example, argues for an understanding of pain as a subjective experience and for the concomitant view of information about pain as falling within the private data domain as opposed to the domain of public data appropriate in the study of phenomena open to direct observation and/or objective measurement.

Others have called for a more radical reformulation of how the person is viewed in clinical practice (Leder, 1984, 1990; Leonard, 1989; Lieb, 1976). These writers argue that both illness and medical practice contribute to a sense of alienation and distancing between the patient and his or her own body and between the patient and the health care providers. What the phenomenological perspective offers is an alternative view of the person and the nature of embodiment. In this context, pain is particularly significant. People in pain cannot escape their own bodies since

> pain, while alienating the self from its corporeality is also...an irrefutable experience of mind-body unity. That the body is not a mere extrinsic machine but our living centre from which radiates all existential possibilities is brought home with a vengeance in illness, suffering, and disability. (Leder, 1984, p. 34)

If this proposition is taken seriously, then studies of patients' experience of pain need to be conducted within a framework that rejects mind-body dualism, with its associated view of the body as an object, and accepts instead the importance of individual and context-specific experience.

In adopting a phenomenological perspective, the present study approaches the question of inflicted pain not as a technical problem in search of a solution, but as a complex human experience to be explored as it is lived. Human life is "complicated, ambiguous, and mysterious" (Munhall, 1989), as are human experiences through which that life is lived.

THE NATURE OF PHENOMENOLOGICAL INQUIRY

The term *phenomenology* is derived from the Greek words *phainomenon* ("an appearance") and *logos* ("word" or "reason," hence "a reasoned inquiry"). Phenomenology, therefore, is a reasoned inquiry into the nature of appearances: appearances referring to anything of which one is conscious (Stewart & Mickunas, 1974, p. 3). Others have defined phenomenology as "a study of essences" (Merleau-Ponty, 1962, p. vii), "essence" referring to the "essential nature" or "that what makes a thing what it is" (van Manen, 1990, p. 177). The distinguishing mark of phenomenology is its primary concern with the nature and meaning of human experience as it is lived. In other words, "phenomenology is the study of the lifeworld," the world of direct experience, with the aim of insightful understanding and description of that experience (van Manen, 1990, p. 9). Furthermore, phenomenology focuses on the study of phenomena not as "objective" entities in and of themselves, but of phenomena as they are perceived or as they are experienced. The aims of phenomenological inquiry are very different from those of natural science. Rather than striving for explanation, prediction and control, phenomenological research aims for an understanding that makes human experience more meaningful and its conceptualization more directly connected to the lived world (Langer, 1989; Reinharz, 1983; van Manen, 1990).

Contemporary phenomenology has its roots in the work of the Viennese philosopher Franz Brentano (1838–1917) and his students, most notably Edmund Husserl (1859–1938). The ground work prepared by Husserl, in turn, paved the way for the early German phase in the development of phenomenology, made prominent in Husserl's own writings as well as those of his one-time assistant, Martin Heidegger (1889–1976). Husserl also provided the stimulus for the later French phase, evidenced in the works of Gabriel Marcel (1889–1973), Jean-Paul Sartre (1905–1980), and particularly Maurice Merleau-Ponty (1908–1961) (Cohen, 1987; Spiegelberg, 1969).

Phenomenology is not a rigidly defined school of thought, and there is considerable diversity in how phenomenology has been used and developed by its major proponents. Most of the early phenomenological writing is concerned with questions of ontology and epistemology, including the issues of existence, consciousness and ultimate meaning (Heidegger, 1962; Marcel, 1960, 1965; Merleau-Ponty, 1962). *Consciousness, perception, embodiment, temporality*, and *experience* as the *being-in-the-world* have come to be regarded as the central concepts of phenomenology as philosophy. The present study uses the work of Merleau-Ponty, and the discussion that follows will focus primarily on his view of phenomenology and ideas about embodiment.

In the preface to his seminal work *The phenomenology of perception*, first published in 1945, Merleau-Ponty presents his most succinct arguments in defense of phenomenology. Using the key themes proposed by Husserl and Heidegger, Merleau-Ponty (1962, p. vii) defines phenomenology as "a study of essences" that requires the researcher return to the reality of the lived world, the world that precedes knowledge and of which knowledge is an abstraction. Thus, Merleau-Ponty makes a fundamental distinction between experience (of movement, pain, or whatever) as it is lived by a person and conceptualizations of human experience abstracted through scientific or other modes of thinking. In making the distinction, Merleau-Ponty is critical of the artificiality and destructiveness of scientific thinking "which looks on from above" (cited in Langer, 1989, p. xi). Instead, he calls for a return to the embodied experience, the prereflective world that people already live before they develop knowledge about it. At the heart of phenomenology, for Merleau-Ponty, is the aim to provide a direct description of human experience as it is for those living the experience and to do so in a rigorous scientific way. In this he is following through with Husserl's phenomenological principle of *returning to things themselves*, of apprehending human experience as it is lived in the context in which it occurs and which it helps to shape:

> To return to things themselves is to return to that world which precedes knowledge, of which knowledge always *speaks*, and in relation to which every scientific schematization is an abstract and derivative sign-language, as is geography in relation to the countryside in which we have learned beforehand what a forest, a prairie or a river is. (Merleau-Ponty, 1962, p. ix)

In her critical assessment of Merleau-Ponty's *Phenomenology of perception*, Langer (1989) suggests that his central concern "is to prompt us to recognize that objective thought fundamentally distorts the phenomena of our lived experience, thereby estranging us from our own selves, the world in which we live and other people with whom we interact" (p. 149). This point is of particular relevance to the study of pain, where scientific research has often objectified the phenomenon of pain and so failed to understand it as it is for those who experience it in their embodied selves. Applying methods of natural science to the study of human life and activity is not only reductionistic, it also produces results that have limited usefulness. The main problem, according to Dreyfus (1984), arises from seeking "a theory that predicts events in the everyday world using context-free features abstracted from that world" (p. 8). Theoretical abstraction removes individual meaning from consideration, and such decontextualization leads to unreliable prediction, thus thwarting one of the central aims of scientific theory: prediction and control. The solution proposed by Dreyfus (1984) is for human sciences to engage in "a disciplined study of human beings which does not seek to be a *theory*, but still seeks to be a systematic account of everyday activities" (p. 16). This is the aim expressed by Merleau-Ponty some 40 years earlier.

What Merleau-Ponty argues for is the notion of *lebenswelt*, the *lifeworld*, proposed earlier by Husserl as the central theme of phenomenology. Human experience, including the experience of pain and suffering, can be understood only when seen in the context of the lifeworld, "a total sphere of experience circumscribed by a natural environment, man-made objects, events, and other individuals" (Wuthnow, Hunter, Bergesen, & Kurzweil, 1984, p. 31), including the personal and cultural situations that give meaning to the experience. These *situated meanings* must be taken into account if the essential nature of particular human experiences is to be understood and described.

Together with the direct experience of the lifeworld, situated meanings give rise to *situated personal knowledge*, which informs us not only about the world, but also about our involvement in that world. The relationship between the person and the situation means that "I am not merely involved in such situations; the situations help to reveal me to myself" (Marcel, 1984a, p. 294). Situated personal knowledge draws on shared meanings and challenges the extremes of both empiricism, which sees knowledge as impersonal, decontextualized and value-free, and subjectivism, which considers it to be value-laden and idiosyncratic (Barratt, 1988; Polanyi, 1958). For Merleau-Ponty, the dichotomy is between the "empiricist or mechanistic psychologies and the intellectualist ones," neither of which he finds adequate for understanding human experience. Like behavior, on which Merleau-Ponty (1965) has written in depth, the experience of pain lies between the traditionally separate mind and body and cannot be adequately accounted for either by the empiricist or the intellectualist schools of thought. To paraphrase Wild (1965), pain is neither a series of blind reactions to external or internal stimuli nor the projection of a disembodied mind. The study of pain has suffered from attempts to explain it scientifically as an essentially bio-physiological event of nociception on the one hand or as an entirely subjective, idiosyncratic experience of suffering on the other.

What phenomenology offers is the possibility of studying human experience, including the experience of pain, in the context of the lifeworld; and therefore, it is able to take into account not only individual meanings of the situation, but also, and more important, the *intersubjectivity* of human experience, the shared meanings that act as a basis for social interaction (Wuthnow et al., 1984). Experience is not something inside the person; rather, "experience is always already out in the world" because the person is always directed toward and involved in the world (Colaizzi, 1978, p. 52). Experience is a mode of presence to the world that is existentially significant and, as such, a legitimate and necessary content for the study of human life and action. Additionally, experience requires involvement from the researcher. As Straus (1966) sums it up, the logico-positivistic approach of traditional science makes the researchers interchangeable but detached from the object of their study since "they all sit in the audience and watch the events on the stage" (p. 259). With human experience, such detachment breaks down as one is drawn into the arena and caught and affected by the experience.

So far the discussion has touched on important phenomenological themes: the lifeworld, personal knowledge, situated meanings, and the inter-subjectivity of human experience in terms of shared experience and meanings. McConville (1978) argues that "for natural science meaning is a sort of embarrassment because it resists reductive causal analysis," while "phenomenology, by contrast, takes meaning as the starting point" (p. 102). Meaning is intrinsic to the human being in the world, and it defines the interface between the person and the lifeworld with which the person is inextricably connected. Phenomenology maintains that meanings are contextually constructed as intersubjective phenomena (Anderson, 1989). In Merleau-Ponty's (1962) words, "Because we are in the world, we are *condemned to meaning*, and we cannot do or say anything without its acquiring a name in history" (p. xix).

Of particular concern to the present study is the account of the lived body as the mode of one's being in the world and the importance of individual experience in our understanding of human life. Merleau-Ponty has developed these themes most clearly in his two early works, *Phenomenology of perception* (1962) and *The structure of behavior* (1965). The importance of individual experience in the study of human life has influenced the design and methods of the present study, while the account of the lived body has provided it with a philosophical orientation and focus and is discussed in the next section.

THE PHENOMENOLOGICAL VIEW OF THE PERSON AND THE CONCEPT OF EMBODIMENT

It has been suggested that the emphasis on the body evident in the works of the early twentieth-century existentialists and phenomenologists arose as a needed corrective to the previous centuries' philosophical preoccupation with abstract reason and the relegation of the body to the status of an object, which, like other objects in nature, could be understood in purely mechanistic terms (Cohen 1984; Stewart & Mickunas, 1974). But the body is not just another rediscovered concern for phenomenological inquiry: it is central to the understanding of human life in the world. In Merleau-Ponty's terms, "To be a body, is to be tied to a certain world....Our body is not primarily *in* space: it is of it" (Merleau-Ponty, 1962, p. 148), just as "the soul remains coextensive with nature" (Merleau-Ponty, 1965, p. 189).

To conceive of the human body as a physical body with measurable properties of mass, weight, size and motion in relation to other objects is to provide only a partial account of its characteristics and activity. Such a view has made possible the many advances in biomedicine and is accepted by phenomenology as valid within its particular sphere of understanding, although it is not considered to have the capacity to provide a complete account of human behavior (Stewart & Mickunas, 1974). To say that the human body is no more than "the assemblage of flesh, bones, and organs which the anatomist anatomizes" and "what the undertakers bury when they bury you" (Campbell, 1984, p. 2) is to ignore embodied intelligence and skills that connect human beings with the world and allow us to inhabit it in a unique way. One's actions, whether speaking, walking, or eating, characterize one's lived body as one's own and no one else's (Merleau-Ponty, 1962). Thus, the lived body communicates a unity and common style of bodily actions that others may observe but which the person experiences as uniquely his or her own (Zaner, 1964). While there is a growing recognition that clinical knowledge, used by nurses and physicians, must include more than just the knowledge of the natural sciences, there is still a tendency to accept the mechanistic model of the person to which is added knowledge from the social sciences and humanities (Bench, 1989).

When the mechanistic view of the person and the nature of embodiment is used as a basis for a study, not of physical objects but of human action and experience, it is not only inadequate, but also confusing and alienating (Benner & Wrubel, 1989). It leads to what Gaines (1985, p. 231) has termed the "referential" or "ego-centric" conception of the person, seen as the dominant ideology in Western medicine. Within it, the person is "a bounded, physical entity; personhood is coterminous with the extent of the physical body, the domain of the core of medicine," and the self is seen as a whole, "complete unto itself" (Gaines, 1985, p. 231). The implication is that illness (including psychiatric illness) is located within the person, that is, within the physical confines of the person, and that medical intervention is a dyadic process between the physician and the patient. Such a view contrasts markedly with the "indexical, socio-centric" conception of the person that Gaines ascribes to the Mediterranean tradition, within which the person is seen to be a spiritual self, integrated into a social and spiritual world: "The self is not solely, or even primarily, a physical entity—a unique, corporeal object. The boundary...is drawn around, or is permeated by extracorporeal elements." A person lacking in spiritual and social integration is by definition "incomplete" and requires healing beyond the domains of internal medicine (Gaines, 1985, pp. 231–232).

Phenomenology has produced proponents of both a theistic (e.g., Marcel) and atheistic position (e.g., Sartre) as well as those like Heidegger (and perhaps Merleau-Ponty) who remained open to either stance. Nevertheless, in placing emphasis on the lived body as a way of understanding one's being in the world, phenomenology is at least in principle closer to the traditional cultural views of the person as embodied spirit than the mechanistic view, which, with its reductionism, dehumanizes that which cannot but be human. In phenomenology, the body is our basic mode of being in the world, consciousness is embodied consciousness, and a person is embodied being, not just the possessor of a body. In phenomenological terms, "one cannot say that *I have a body* or even *I am a body*, but rather *I am bodily* as incarnate subjectivity" (Stewart & Mickunas, 1974, p. 66).

Any study of human existence must have a starting point of which it is certain, a point of departure from which to explore that about which it is not certain. For phenomenology, particularly as developed by Marcel and Merleau-Ponty, that point of departure is "the immediacy of lived existence," and the body, the "incarnate being," is "the touchstone of existence" (Straus & Machado, 1984, p. 123). The phenomenological idea of the *lived body* goes much further than the concepts of "body-image," "body-schema," or "somatognosis" found in the literature on psychology and neurology, and which attempts to unite the mind and the body within the pre-existing frameworks (Moss, 1978, p. 75). One underlying assumption in the use of such terms is that we perceive our own bodies in basically the same detached way that we may employ when viewing any other object outside of ourselves.

The "constancy hypothesis" is another assumption of the traditional scientific view of how people perceive changes within their own bodies. The hypothesis is that there is a one-to-one correspondence between a sensory stimulus and the resulting "objective" sensation felt by the individual. When distortion of this primary correspondence occurs, which it frequently does, it is said to be brought about by a secondary process of subjective interpretation and the addition of meanings independent of the original stimulus (Moss, 1978).

Both of the above assumptions have significant implications for the study and understanding of pain. In this context, the constancy hypothesis has been challenged, most cogently by the formulation of the gate-control theory of pain (Melzack & Wall, 1965, 1988), and yet it underlies much of the laboratory research on pain. The specific assumption is that experimentally produced and therefore highly measurable stimulus for pain will produce a corresponding level of physical pain, without the contaminating influences of other factors present in pain associated with illness or injury (Over, 1980). Even in clinical settings, the extent of tissue damage is frequently regarded as the prime indicator of how much pain a patient should be experiencing or expressing at a particular time (Madjar, 1981). As already discussed earlier in this chapter, correlational studies of patients following burn injuries continue to look for predictable relationships between the extent of injury and the amount of pain patients are likely to experience, even though the research evidence does not support the hypothesis for such a correlation.

In his writings, Merleau-Ponty (1962) argues against both the idea of an objective approach to the knowledge of the embodied self and the constancy hypothesis. He consistently returns to the primacy of existence within which we do not so much *know* our bodies as *live* them. In the words of another phenomenologist,

> Prior to *reflecting* on our bodies and prior to *knowing* about our bodies, we live our bodies and develop our bodies' capacity for action. In so doing we build up a *lived* familiarity with the body as a vehicle for action. (Moss, 1978, pp. 75–76)

In making his stand, Merleau-Ponty (1962) does not reject the presence of the material, anatomical body, understood through "mechanistic physiology" and able to be seen as a mere physical object. His argument is that the "res extensa," the object-body of Descartes, is a derivative, arising out of the experience of the lived body (Leder, 1984). It is also a constructed representation that, while necessary in understanding a particular level of physiological function, provides an inadequate basis for understanding a person's behavior, experience or expressions.

Even though, as Leder (1990) points out, it is the material body that the physician examines and to which the treatment is directed, *my* experience of *my* body is of a different order. In support of his argument, Merleau-Ponty points to the experience of pain as something that happens not to an object, however close to the essential self, but rather within the very fabric of one's being:

> For if I say that my foot hurts, I do not simply mean that it is a cause of pain in the same way as the nail which is cutting into it, differing only in being nearer to me; I do not mean that it is the last of the objects in the external world, after which a more intimate kind of pain should begin, an unlocalized awareness of pain in itself, related to the foot only by some causal connection and within the closed system of experience. I mean that the pain reveals itself as localized, that it is constitutive of a "pain-infested space." "My foot hurts" means not: "I think that my foot is the cause of this pain," but: "the pain comes from my foot" or again "my foot has a pain." (Merleau-Ponty, 1962, p. 93)

Thus, there is an inherent uniqueness in how people experience their own bodies for themselves that is different from how they experience external objects. It is this sense of personal integrity, of knowing oneself as uniquely self, that may be disturbed in situations of illness, disability, or unrelieved pain: "In illness the body is experienced as at once intimately mine but also other than-me, in that there is a sense in which I am at its disposal or mercy" (Toombs, 1987, p. 230).

In the context of painful or embarrassing physical examinations, patients may experience and seek an attitude of detachment as a way of coping with the impact of disruption to their habitual being in the world. While helpful in the short-term, such detachment can lead to the experience of dehumanization, whether directed toward oneself or toward others (Bernard, Ottenberg, & Redl, 1977). Dehumanization involves a decreased sense of one's own individuality and of the humanness of others. In clinical settings, staff may also try to cope in stressful situations by viewing others, temporarily perhaps, as inanimate objects on which tasks such as dressing changes need to be accomplished. The paradox in such a situation is that even while treating another as an objective body a nurse (or a physician) continues to be (that is, to experience him/herself as) a lived body, relying on skilled actions and his/her own embodied intelligence. As Straus (1984) points out, a physician does not see his or her hands as bones and tendons or eyes as cornea and retina as he or she sees the corresponding organs of the patient: "The doctor remains a paradigmatic instance of the lived body in praxis" (p. 34). So even as we succeed in seeing the other as an objective body of anatomical structures and physiological functions, we continue to experience ourselves in quite a different way.

Phenomenological account of the lived body

Merleau-Ponty's account of the *lived body* aims to understand the body as one lives and experiences it as opposed to the body known by natural science or disinterested observation. The lived body is "not just a caused mechanism, but an *intentional* entity always directed toward an object pole, a world" (Leder, 1984, p. 31). Merleau-Ponty himself seldom uses the term lived body and does not present an exposition of its different facets in a clear, organized fashion; rather, he keeps returning to the body in various contexts and revealing aspects of it that together add up to an account of the lived body.

Benner and Wrubel (1989, p. 70) provide one of the clearest and for the present study most relevant summaries of Merleau-Ponty's account of embodiment, which is based on Hubert Dreyfus' unpublished work. They identify five dimensions of the lived body, the "me as incarnate subject" (Merleau-Ponty, 1962, p. 52): the inborn complex; the habitual, skilled body; the projective body; the actual projected body; and the phenomenal body.

The inborn complex describes the prepersonal, precultural body existing even in utero but which already has skills such as thumb sucking and turning in response to light or sound. Even as we develop, we retain something of this inborn complex, which even though precultural "is not some kind of inert thing; it too has something of the momentum of existence" (Merleau-Ponty, 1962, p. 84).

The habitual, skilled body describes the socially and culturally acquired postures, gestures and habits that allow the person to share the world with others. The habitual, skilled body develops through imitation and practice rather than through didactic instruction. Benner and Wrubel (1989, p. 71) give the example of the culture-specific behaviors in relation to personal space and social distance. Americans, Mexicans or Japanese normally observe quite definite customs in terms of how close they will stand to others in different situations, and yet they would find it difficult to specify the appropriate distances in terms of inches or centimeters.

Skill acquisition is another example of the habitual body, whether the skill is swimming, riding a bicycle, or performing an intricate nursing procedure. Normally such embodied skills are put into action smoothly and without conscious effort. However, difficulties may arise when the "habit-body" is in contradiction to the "body at this moment" (Merleau-Ponty, 1962, p. 82), for example, in the case of amputation. The person whose arm has been amputated may reach to grasp an object only to find that the arm he/she experiences as reaching out is in fact not there. The persistence of the habitual body cannot be accounted for in terms of simple memory and imagination:

> The phantom arm is not a recollection, it is a quasi-present and the patient feels it now, folded over his chest, with no hint of its belonging to the past. Nor can we suppose that the image of an arm, wondering through consciousness, has joined itself to the stump: For then it would not be a "phantom," but a renascent perception. The phantom arm must be that same arm, lacerated by shell splinters, its visible substance burned or rotted somewhere, which appears to haunt the present body without being absorbed into it. (Merleau-Ponty, 1962, p. 85)

Difficulties may also arise when the sense of the habitual body is altered or temporarily lost, as in the following example. Oliver Sacks (1984) gives a vivid personal account of recovery from a leg injury: despite his surgeon's assurances that he should be able to do so, he found himself unable to walk on a leg that felt alien and out of his control. Verbal instructions and conscious effort produced no results until pushed into a swimming pool and challenged to race. At that point the habitual body took over and he swam and, once out of the pool, walked without difficulty. Injury or illness can lead to a loss of a person's habitual body, making the body feel strange and distant: "Without a habitual, skilled body, people find all activity effortful and deliberate" (Benner & Wrubel, 1989, p. 73).

The projective body describes the way the body is set to move or act in everyday life, for example, when reaching for an object or performing a skilled manoeuvre. This requires more than just eye and hand coordination; it demonstrates "a unity of sensory-motor intentionality" (Leder, 1984, p. 37), that is, without thinking one knows how far to reach or how to retain balance. For Merleau-Ponty (1962, p. 149), this is not a question of "simple," learned coordination of the body's visual, tactile, and motor aspects but rather the projection of the body toward a goal that connects various aspects into a "common meaning." The projective body can be affected by illness, for example, when a person trying to make the first step after a period of immobilization has to visually locate the affected leg and consciously calculate where and how to move it (Sacks, 1984, p. 104). The difficulties associated with achieving coordinated movement through conscious effort during rehabilitation are a useful reminder of the extent to which the projected body is taken for granted in everyday life.

The actual projected body describes "one's current actual projection" (Benner & Wrubel, 1989, p. 74) or a complex of projected bodily skills related to a particular activity, such as driving a car. A good example is a nurse administering intravenous chemotherapy and attending both to the physical procedure and the patient's response, "feeling" the patient's tension build up or recede and adjusting the procedure and his/her communication with the patient accordingly.

The phenomenal body describes "the body aware of itself" (Benner & Wrubel, 1989, p. 75), including bodily sensations and body image. The phenomenal body can be experienced in relation to bodily sensations, for example, pain during labor and birthing. Such pain can be experienced and described in very personal ways, for example, as good, bearable, or overwhelming, as well as "objectively," for example, as a series of contractions of certain frequency, duration and intensity. The phenomenal body can also be experienced through culturally developed ways, such as the knowledge of human anatomy. It is thus possible for people to imagine specific organs within their own bodies and through the techniques of biofeedback and visualization to have some, albeit limited influence on certain bodily functions (Benner & Wrubel, 1989). The phenomenal body may also be extended beyond its anatomical boundaries, for example, when a blind person uses a stick so that it becomes "an extension of the bodily synthesis," and "the world of feelable things recedes and now begins, not at the outer skin of the hand, but at the end of the stick" (Merleau-Ponty, 1962, p. 152).

In health, we experience our embodied selves in an unself-conscious way, taking for granted and paying little attention to processes such as breathing or the position of our limbs in relation to the rest of the body. In illness, one's own body can no longer be taken for granted. There is a breakdown, a discontinuity in one's being in the world as pain, dyspnoea, nausea or other sensations draw attention to themselves and to the body and make one's being in the world unpredictable and effortful. When the disability is chronic or progressive, the person may experience a kind of disembodiment that can totally change his or her sense of place in the world, and yet, as the following extract from Murphy (1987) illustrates, health professionals show little interest in the person's lived experience and therefore continue to act on the basis of information that does not include the patient's understanding of the situation:

> From the time my tumor was first diagnosed through my entry into wheelchair life, I had an increasing apprehension that I had lost much more than the full use of my legs. I had also lost a part of myself. It was not just that people acted differently toward me, which they did,

but rather that I felt differently toward myself. I had changed in my own mind, in my self-image, and in the basic conditions of my existence. It left me feeling alone and isolated, despite strong support from family and friends.

Nobody has ever asked me what it is like to be a paraplegic—and now a quadriplegic—for this would violate all the rules of middle-class etiquette....Polite manners may protect us from most such intrusions, but it is remarkable that physicians seldom ask either. They like "hard facts" obtainable through modern technology or old-fashioned jabbing with a pin and asking whether you feel it. These tests supposedly provide good, "objective" measures of neurological damage, but, like sociological questionnaires, they reduce experience to neat distinctions of black or white and ignore the broad range of ideation and emotion that always accompanies disability.

I have also become rather emotionally detached from my body, often referring to one of my limbs as *the* leg or *the* arm....As my condition has deteriorated, I have come increasingly to look upon my body as a faulty life-support system, the only function of which is to sustain my head. (Murphy, 1987, pp. 85–101)

People who experience a sense of disembodiment as a result of disease or injury may need help in becoming reembodied into a body that is phenomenally as well as objectively different (Williams, 1984). Others, such as Robert Murphy, cited above, may need assistance in adjusting to a life of permanent disembodiment when the anatomical body may be intact (although its physiological functions might be impaired) but the habitual-skilled and the projective body are lost and the phenomenal body altered beyond anything one has previously known. The title of Murphy's (1987) book, *The body silent*, captures the depth of estrangement experienced by a person who has over time become quadriplegic.

Embodiment and pain

Pain has a different impact on the embodied self. There is no bodily silence in pain. Addis (1986) suggests that pain imposes its presence, requiring one's attention, not only by its intensity, but also, as Merleau-Ponty (1962) has indicated, by its spatiality—it is always located in a certain place in the body.

In her treatise on the vulnerability of the human body and the political consequences of deliberately inflicted pain, Elaine Scarry (1985) identifies some of the essential qualities of pain and their impact on the person in pain and on others. First, there is the quality of invisibility and inexplicability about pain that makes it possible for a person to be physically near someone in pain and not be aware of the pain. Unlike other states of consciousness, bodily pain has no outside point of reference, no referential content. It just is: "It is not *of* or *for* anything. It is precisely because it takes no object that it, more than any other phenomenon, resists objectification in language" (Scarry, 1985, p. 5). Marcel (1984b, p. 335) also speaks of the "uncommunicable aspect" of pain that may contribute to feelings of not only being threatened, but also of being trapped in a hurting body that has taken on the role of a master.

Second, because bodily pain resists objectification in language, this contributes to its unsharability. In other words, pain actively destroys language, one of the culturally learned ways of being in the world with others. The reversion to a prelanguage state of cries and moans signifies destruction of language, but it also signifies destruction of the person's habitual and projective body and a profound change in the phenomenal body. Scarry (1985) argues for a need to have others speak on behalf of those in pain who are unable to speak for themselves. There are, however, many impediments to expressing another's distress, one of the most important being the inability or unwillingness to hear the expression of pain from the person in pain. Health professionals may not trust patient's expressions of pain and may

> perceive the voice of the patient as an "unreliable narrator" of bodily events, a voice which must be by-passed as quickly as possible so that they can get around and behind it to the physical events themselves. But if the only external sign of the felt-experience of pain…is the patient's verbal report…then to by-pass the voice is to by-pass the bodily event, to by-pass the patient, to by-pass the person in pain. (Scarry, 1985, pp. 6–7)

The other side of this picture is that in order to gain control over pain it is necessary to give it voice so that its verbal expression serves as a prelude to the shared project of reducing pain.

The third point relates to the way "pain enters our midst as at once something that cannot be denied and something that cannot be confirmed." It is precisely because we know our own bodies in a way that is fundamentally different from the way we know anyone else's body that "to have pain is to have *certainty*; to hear about pain is to have *doubt*" (Scarry, 1985, p. 13).

The issues raised by Scarry (1985) and the preceding discussion argue that pain needs to be understood in its lived, embodied context. Similarly, in clinical practice, it is not enough to attend to the anatomical body or to a person's "psychological needs" alone. It is the lived body in all its dimensions, the incarnate person who needs attention and care. Such care cannot be based on scientific knowledge alone; it must include a phenomenological understanding of human experience and its individual and shared meanings. A phenomenological understanding cannot be gained by using the methods of traditional science but by using its own methods and procedures. Merleau-Ponty (1962) puts it unequivocally when he states that "phenomenology is accessible only through a phenomenological method" (p. viii).

NURSING AND PHENOMENOLOGY

Gadow (1980) suggests that in its early days nursing, in its concern with the immediate comfort of the patient, focused on the lived body. This perspective was lost, however, when the concern shifted to the biophysiological condition of the patient, with its focus on the objective body. Nursing scholars have questioned this shift in perspective and argued that nursing needs frameworks of nursing practice and knowledge organization. Contemporary statements on nursing illustrate the reformulated core values of the discipline when they stress that nursing is concerned with the human experiences of health and illness rather than treatment of disease (Benner, 1985), human capacities for ongoing self-care necessary for health maintenance and restoration (Orem, 1985), and "caring for those who need to be nurtured in relation to their health status" (Styles, 1982, p. 230).

Earlier definitions of *man* as a bio-psycho-social being (e.g., Roy, 1976) are being replaced with definitions of the *person* as an interconnected energy field (Newman, 1986), an experiencing subject characterized by a pattern and interrelated with the environment (Parse, 1987), and the Hiedeggerian views of the person as a self-interpreting, embodied intelligence, situated in a world and concerned in it (Benner & Wrubel, 1989; Leonard, 1989). Predating these developments has been nursing's belief that understanding the patients' perspectives on their experience of health and illness is a key prerequisite to optimal nursing care (Orlando, 1961; Travelbee, 1971). Leininger (1978) and others also claim that it is important to understand the patient's cultural background and perspectives.

All of these developments, together with the growing recognition of the inadequacies of the biomedical model as a sole basis for *nursing* practice, make links between nursing and phenomenology both possible and understandable. Phenomenology provides nursing with a richer, more adequate philosophical basis for understanding the human experiences of health, illness, disability, coping, recovery, and endurance in the face of ongoing difficulties and suffering. The phenomenological perspective on the person is compatible with the growing concern in nursing to address itself to whole persons within their social and cultural environments. Such a perspective also offers a new understanding and appreciation of skilled nursing practices, which have gone unrecognized or unvalued within the dominant biomedical model (Benner, 1984a; Benner & Tanner, 1987). More visibly, as nurses have collectively come to view themselves as belonging to a professional discipline responsible for the development of its own body of knowledge, phenomenology has contributed significantly to the development and conduct of nursing research and scholarly writing (e.g., Benner, 1984a; Benner & Wrubel, 1989; Gadow, 1984; Sandelowski & Pollock, 1986).

Along with other forms of qualitative research, phenomenological methods have contributed to a growing body of nursing research that adds to our understanding of the patients' lived experience: for example, the experience of courage in the context of life-threatening illness (Haase, 1987); women's experiences of infertility and related treatment (Sandelowski & Pollock, 1986); women's experiences of living with breast cancer (Kesselring, 1990); and the development of the early phases of attachment between mothers and their infants (Stainton, 1985). Others have used the phenomenological perspective to examine the transformation of women to mothers (Bergum, 1989), work-related stress and coping in mid-career men (Benner, 1984b), the practice-embedded knowledge of nurses and the domains and nature of their work (Benner, 1984a), the use of therapeutic touch in nursing practice (Lionberger, 1985), and the structure of caring interactions in nursing (Riemen, 1986b). Such studies are important beyond their immediate illumination of the issues under study. Free of the constraints and assumptions of the quantitative approach, phenomenological research in nursing has asked hitherto unasked questions and produced descriptions and interpretations, exemplars and paradigm cases that depict the reality of human experience and nursing practice in a way that statistical manipulation of values assigned to operationally defined variables cannot do. Such research speaks to nurses in clinical practice as much as it speaks to other researchers and scholars, and this is one of its major strengths. Referring to qualitative research generally, Swanson and Chenitz (1982) sum up the situation when they say that

> qualitative research provides a way to construct meaning that is more reflective of the world of practice because its methodology, like its

subject, is more organic than mechanistic and, therefore, more suitable to the study of the domain of professional nursing. (p. 245)

In turn, it needs to be noted that phenomenological research in nursing is making its contributions to phenomenology. The lived body and the life-world are not the same in health as in illness, crisis, or transition into motherhood. The alteration or loss of one's usual being in the world and the communication of such experiences to others can deepen our understanding of human life, coping and healing. Nurse researchers, with their wealth of contextual knowledge and understanding of illness and health care institutions, are uniquely placed to conduct phenomenological studies where other researchers may be unacceptable to the participants or unable to develop the necessary quality of dialogue with them (Reinharz, 1983).

Despite the growing recognition of its strengths, phenomenological research in nursing is not without its critics. There are many who see it as inferior or at best preliminary to experimental research. When such views are held by those who assess applications for research funding or control access to potential research settings or scholarly publications, nurses wishing to undertake qualitative research may face discouragement and practical difficulties. Skepticism about the ability of phenomenological research to achieve some of its major claims has also been expressed. Salsberry (1989), for example, questions the claims that "understanding an experience of some concept like health or courage will uncover knowledge of the essential structure of the concept" or that "understanding the experience of a concept is useful and important for the generation of knowledge" (p. 10). Such criticisms are productive in that they require proponents of phenomenological research to clarify their thinking and to justify the stand they take. Smith (1989), in responding directly to Salsberry, accepts the usefulness of her criticism but also points out the inappropriateness of evaluating phenomenology from within the framework of traditional positivist science. More specifically, she cites Merleau-Ponty's argument that knowledge is mediated by experience and that the richness and complexity of human experience has primacy over theoretical frameworks in the development of knowledge.

When research questions relate to human experiences and the meanings such experiences have for the people involved (questions that lie at the heart of nursing), then the phenomenological approach has much to offer. As more phenomenological research is undertaken in nursing, its potential and significance for nursing practice and education will become more evident. The present study is a contribution toward that goal.

Chapter 3
Placing the Experience of Inflicted Pain in Context: The Impact of Illness and Injury on the Embodied Self

The nature and aims of phenomenology are concerned with understanding human experiences in their contexts and their complexity. Thus, the need to consider the context of the experience of inflicted pain is an integral part of phenomenological inquiry. What constitutes the context of a particular experience, however, can be open to debate. The research on which this book is based began with the idea that the physical and social environment of the hospital, the presence of illness and injuries, the impact of treatment, and the concerns about recovery might be important facets of the context in which patients experience inflicted pain. In many respects, these factors are relevant to the aim of understanding in context. I also commenced the research aware of the centrality of the idea of embodiment in the phenomenology of Merleau-Ponty and its potential significance for understanding human pain. However, it was only later, in the process of reflection on some of the early findings, that I became aware of the connections between patients' experiences of changes to their embodied selves and what, for them, constituted the context of their lived experiences. In other words, clinically inflicted pain affects people already unsettled by changes brought about by illness or injury, people who may be hurting, scared, confused, or angry, people who for a time at least have lost the taken-for-granted familiarity with their own bodies.

To understand inflicted pain, therefore, it is necessary to understand the context of changed embodiment in which the experience is situated and which helps to give rise to meanings that come to exemplify the experience. There are two main themes that describe the patients' experience of changes to their embodied being as the context for their experience of clinically inflicted pain: *losing a sense of the habitual body* through the impact of illness, injury, and the experience of diagnostic and treatment procedures and *regaining one's habitual body* in the midst of a difficult personal situation.

THE SIGNIFICANCE OF THE CONTEXT

It is possible to focus on pain as a particular phenomenon. However, the experience of having cancer and receiving chemotherapy or being burned and needing to have dressing changes involves a great deal more than being in pain. In the writing of this book, it has been necessary to be constantly attentive to the balance between figure (pain) and ground (the broader experience of injury/illness and treatment). Too great a stress on pain would decontextualize it and make its meanings more difficult to grasp. Similarly, too much emphasis on the broader experience of illness and treatment could result in an inadequate explication of the phenomenon of pain, thereby jeopardizing the overall aim of achieving a deeper understanding of what it is to experience inflicted pain.

The context of an experience may have many facets, from the physical location and facilities to the organizational setting and the network of professional and social relationships that give the place a particular atmosphere or "sentimental order" (Fagerhaugh & Strauss, 1977, p. 290). Some of the physical features had a profound effect on the patients' experience. For example, the contrast between the comfort and familiarity of their own homes and the very different atmosphere and strangeness of the hospital laboratory and clinic rooms was felt very keenly by patients with cancer. The hospital environment, which they experienced in relatively brief episodes, remained a hated place, which not only looked, felt, and smelled in a way that was discomforting, but was a (literally) concrete witness to what was wrong with them and why they had to come within its confines. At home, they could feel stronger connections to their old selves; in hospital, everything was a reminder of their illness and of their changed and precarious being-in-the-world.

Initially, at least, patients with burns had a different response to the hospital environment. The suddenness and severity of their injuries made them feel a need for comfort and protection. The isolation room, with its temperature and humidity controls, where they were allowed to rest after initial assessment and treatment, quickly became a haven, a place of safety. The eventual move out into the ward and into the company of other patients was seen as a first step in returning to the social world as a changed person, and patients commented on their reluctance to leave the safety of the isolation room and face others at a time when their burn wounds were far from healed. Even the noise and the general busyness of the normal hospital ward was unsettling and something to which patients needed to adjust.

On the other hand, there were aspects of the environment that gave rise to very similar concerns for both groups of patients. Whenever they were deprived of a view of the world beyond the room in which they were being treated,[1] for example, patients receiving chemotherapy as well as those with burns described feeling *closed in, hot, claustrophobic* and finding it difficult to stay still and allow nurses to complete a procedure. In other words, patients expressed a bodily need to retain at least a visual contact with the world beyond the confining boundaries of the hospital.

It was evident that even the physical environment, as experienced by the patients, was not static but changed depending on whether patients were waiting for treatment, undergoing a diagnostic or treatment procedure, or able to see the outside world during procedures. Those receiving chemotherapy, for example, often described the ambient temperature of the treatment room as *hot* at the end of treatment, even though, while there may have been a change in the patient's body temperature, the temperature of the room itself did not alter.

Organizational aspects of the hospital setting also had an important bearing on the patients' experience. Ward routines in the Burn Care Unit, for example, included not only set meal times, visiting hours, and "wake-up" and "lights-out" times, but also set times for "drug rounds" when pain medication was offered and set "medical rounds" when wound dressings had to be removed so that surgeons could assess healing and readiness for grafting. Having one's wounds unwrapped for a prolonged period of time was an important source of inflicted pain for the patients and is discussed in more detail in the next chapter. The point being made here is that many aspects of the hospital environment contributed to the patients' experience of pain. Infliction of pain was influenced not only by the direct actions of individual nurses or other staff, but also by bureaucratic routines that sometimes dictated the timing of particular procedures or how they would be performed.

Many aspects of the environment, therefore, can affect the patient's experience of pain. And yet, however important they might be, they are largely external to the person, who may have little understanding of their outworkings. The most intimate context of the patients' experience of inflicted pain is not the physical environment of spaces, views, sounds and smells, nor even the social environment of hospital staff, other patients, family members and visitors. The most intimate context of the patient's experience is the changes in the embodied self resulting from the disease or injury that is present within the body of the person and with which he or she must live. The changes brought about by cancer or burns relate to pain in at least two different ways.

First, bodily changes *predicate pain* since without them pain would not occur, and there would be no need for diagnostic and treatment procedures that cause inflicted pain. It was the threat to their bodily integrity that led the patients in the study to seek professional help, so it is something of an irony that in seeking to preserve their intactness they in fact exposed themselves to invasive and painful procedures. This was especially evident in the experience of patients with cancer and is discussed further in the next chapter.

Second, bodily changes brought about by cancer or burns also *situate pain* into a body that is not the normal, familiar body the person knows and through which he or she knows the world. From a situation in which the body is taken for granted, ignored in terms of its anatomical structures, and simply lived, the person is placed in a situation of turning from the world of everyday concerns and social life to becoming aware of a body that is a source of unpleasant and worrying sensations, that does not behave in predictable ways, and that may threaten one's very existence. For a number of the patients in the study, the change in their sense of embodiment was so profound that they felt confused and lost within their own bodies and even estranged from them for a time. It was these immediate concerns that provided the context within which patients experienced pain and within which they had to learn to endure it, come to terms with how it affected them, and find meaning in the experience.

The people affected by cancer or burn injuries must deal with a loss of their *habitual bodies*, the sense of dis-ease that the loss brings, and with the attempts, not always successful, to regain what they had lost and become themselves again. The remainder of this chapter, therefore, deals with the impact of illness and injury on the embodied self, and it explores what it means to be burned or to have cancer and to live through the experience of diagnosis and therapy.

LOSING A SENSE OF THE HABITUAL BODY

To an observer, being burned or having cancer may appear to be two totally different types of experience, and in many ways they are. Cancer often develops very slowly and manifests itself ambiguously. Its diagnosis may require an extensive investigation and may be made only by specially trained physicians. Burn injuries are different. They occur suddenly, and the surface damage is visible to anyone who observes the exposed wounds. Just as important, the pain of burns leaves the injured person in no doubt about the facticity of physical damage and the need for professional help. By contrast, patients with cancer may experience considerable difficulty apprehending the nature of their disease, and they may have doubts about the appropriateness or adequacy of the treatment they are given. The nature of burns and cancer therapies, their frequency and overall duration, and their impact on the people receiving them are all different. So are the possible outcomes.

Nevertheless, the experience-as-lived (whether of burns or cancer) is different from the experience-as-observed, and as different patients' experiences were examined, a strong common thread emerged, as well as, some contrasts. Thus, while outwardly the two groups of patients seemed to have little in common, in terms of their lived experience they shared many common concerns and meanings. The common thread that brought these two kinds of experiences together was the patients' changed sense of embodiment. For the patients, this change occurred when the familiar and taken-for-granted body was changed into something that looked, felt, and was different, an object that was strange and discomforting. Individual experiences may have been outwardly different, but underlying them all was a sense of loss of one's former self, of feeling strange, confused, and not oneself as well as an inability to grasp the full impact of what had happened. In all cases, the changed sense of embodiment began with an awareness of something being wrong.

Sensing that something is wrong

Sensing that something is wrong was the first step on the way toward the diagnosis of cancer. Patients were often struck by the insidious and subtle nature of the initial symptoms and the almost accidental discovery of something out of the ordinary. A person may have started feeling tired and only gradually become aware that the tiredness was not related to daily activities and exertions. Or a lump, a swelling, or a small nodule was noticed while doing nothing more than scratching one's neck or having a shower. Becoming aware that the lump was not there the week before and should not be there now, that the tiredness felt different and *wrong* gave rise to anxiety and a search for explanation. For some, the awareness of something out of the ordinary led to immediate action:

I was scratching my neck and I suddenly felt this lump. I thought that was a bit unusual. That was Sunday night, so I rang the doctor the next day.

For others, there was a considerable delay before seeking medical advise. Eventually (in one case a year after first becoming aware of something being wrong), medical contact was established and the *something wrong* was given a name. However slow and insidious in its development, once named for what it was, cancer assumed a personal reality and presence for these patients. It was no longer something that happened to other people; the cancer was inside them, enmeshed in the very fabric of their bodies and threatening even their survival. From that point on, they could no longer take their bodies for granted. Something was *very wrong*, and the diagnosis of cancer seemed to remove a sense of previously felt mastery over their lives. The knowledge that they had cancer created a rift between themselves as persons and the lives they could see themselves living in the world. They had lost charge of their lives and the ability to influence their future. One young man expressed his loss quietly, with a note of despair in his voice:

I've always been in control of my whole life, up until last October [when cancer was diagnosed], and whatever has gone on in my life has been my doing. I feel, from now on, apart from following instructions, there is nothing; I am not in control of it any more.

All of the patients in this study had known the responsibilities involved in making life-changing decisions (to divorce, to migrate to New Zealand, to adopt a child, to start a new business venture). In acting on such decisions, they felt that they had actively created different possibilities for their being in the world. Receiving a diagnosis of cancer shattered their sense of ability to shape the world around them and thus their own lives. To have their sense of mastery reduced to the choice to follow or not follow others' instructions was to feel a hitherto unknown and profound sense of helplessness, which for some patients persisted throughout their time on chemotherapy.

For patients who suffered burn trauma, *sensing that something was wrong* happened instantaneously and called for the immediate bodily response of getting away from the source of trauma and obtaining help. *Sensing that something was wrong*, however, did not mean that these people were immediately aware either of the nature or the full extent of their injuries. They were aware that their bodies hurt and were strangely unfamiliar. A driver injured while pushing his way out of a burning petrol tanker captured this sense of unfamiliarity as he recalled running across a field toward a farm house and catching the sight of his hands:

> Looking like the blue gum trees...the bark that hangs off, that's what they looked like....[At the same time his hands felt extremely cold]...colder than having your hands nailed into a freezer...extremely painful.

The feeling of *something wrong* was particularly distressing for patients who because of facial burns and swollen eyelids could not see and thus visually check out the nature and extent of their injuries. They could see neither their changed bodies nor the people and activities going on around them. The extreme pain they felt was frightening, and they took it as an indication of extensive bodily damage—the sort of damage that threatened their sense of intactness and created fears of a mutilated appearance. At the same time, while feeling an almost overwhelming need for human comfort and care, it was difficult for them to apprehend what was being done to help them and to feel that they were being given the kind of help they needed. A young woman who suffered an epileptic seizure while getting into a shower and woke up screaming for help following hot water burns to 15 percent of her body provides a vivid description of her distress and others' actions that did not match her felt needs:

> With the ambulance driver, that was really frustrating because I can remember him there, calling, calling me by my name...and telling me that it was going to be all right and that we were on our way to hospital....It must have been just in the way that he was talking or in what he was saying. It just wasn't getting through, and nothing, nothing he said had any soothing effect at all.

(Why do you think that was?)

> I don't think he knew what to do. I don't, I really don't! I don't think he knew or understood the sort of pain I was in, or shock....I don't know if I was crying at that stage, but I was groaning and moaning, yes, possibly crying at that stage....If he had given me his hand, for instance...if I could have just held his hand, but all I could hear was this voice around me. I couldn't see anything, but I could just hear this voice. I really needed something to grasp....I reached a point where I became scared of even wanting to look at my own body because I was scared of what it looked like.

Like patients with cancer, those with burns eventually faced the medical diagnosis and its implications: in their case the need for hospitalization, for grafting surgery, and for coming to terms with a body that had suddenly changed and might never look the way it had looked before being injured.

Sensing that something was wrong was the first indication experienced by both groups of patients of a breakdown, a discontinuity in their being in the world, and a loss of predictability and mastery over their own bodies and their lives. Their bodies were not only objectively different, in terms of neoplastic changes in diseased cells and tissues or the necrotic and inflammatory processes brought about by burns, they were also phenomenally different, feeling discomfort, pain, unease, and many other new and unfamiliar sensations where only a short time before there had been an unself-conscious, taken-for-granted sense of embodiment and being in the world. *Sensing that something was wrong* prompted these people to seek help and in turn helped to make acceptable the diagnostic and treatment procedures they had to undergo. Yet the experience of these same diagnostic and treatment procedures also reinforced for them the feelings of being changed and being different.

Looking different to oneself and to the world

By their very nature burn injuries destroy skin integrity; they create visible wounds and alter a person's appearance. First-degree burns may heal spontaneously and without obvious scarring, while deeper burns may require grafting, which leaves its own kind of scarring and disfigurement. This is the kind of information that patients with burns acquired only gradually and had to learn to accept as knowledge relevant to their own situation. The lived experience of being burned, however, involved *looking different* and, for individual patients at different stages of recovery, *looking bad, not nice, horrible*, and above all *not myself*.

All patients expressed some concern about their appearance and how others would react to it. Those with burns to parts of the body that could be easily covered with clothing expressed relief that their scars would not be readily obvious to others. Often, this was the only indication they gave of being concerned about the way their bodies looked. The expectation that they would appear unchanged to others, however, underscored their unease with how others would have reacted to their marred appearance if the burns had been more extensive or more visible.

In some cases, the possibility of visible scarring threatened a person's cultural identity. A young Maori man, for example, made the following comment when, seeing himself in the mirror for the first time, he noticed patches of new skin on his face:

> I don't like losing my nice Maori skin and have this pink stuff growing. I don't like my face to be pink. I want it nice and brown.

Looking different to oneself and others was an experience that brought some patients to the verge of despair. Initially, they hoped that it was all a bad dream from which they would wake up. It took them weeks to accept that their injuries would not vanish and that they would be left with permanent scars. The experience, however, went deeper than a matter of appearance. Coming to terms with a strange, disfigured, hurting body was not easy. The wounding was not momentary; it was something that came to permeate their whole being, preventing them from feeling at ease in their embodied selves:

> I try and put a patch on it. I try and imagine that it's not there, or it's not really as bad as it looks....Sometimes I wish I couldn't see it, but no, I would rather be able to see what's happened....Sometimes I just look at it and it's almost as if...my other eye which isn't open yet, it's almost a blindfold, too. But I imagine when it's open that the full reality of it will be right there in front of me, but it's almost as if I had this [pointing to the sutured eyelid] as a blindfold, too....I don't really feel that this is part of my body in a way. This is something else, and Geraldine will be Geraldine as she was on Friday in a few weeks.
>
> (But this is not Geraldine?)
>
> No! No, this is another body.
>
> (Another body?)
>
> Mm. This is another body that I don't know. Not me. I don't deserve it. It's not me. I don't deserve it. I've been saying that to myself all day. And I was hoping that it will go away.

Two weeks later this young woman was still struggling to come to terms with the changes that her body had gone through. As she considered the day she would eventually leave the hospital, there were feelings of vulnerability in relation to how she *looked to others* and how they would respond to her marred appearance. The most difficult part of what she tried hard to come to terms with, however, was a deep sense of *alienation from her own disfigured body* and a sense of *loss of her former self.*

> I think I would have been quite happy with all the grafting on my body except my head. I think to lose my hair has been quite upsetting for me…and so I have found it very difficult to come to terms with that over the last few days….The skin has been able to be replaced and the hair can't be replaced, and that's what I feel angry about. I liked my hair….I looked in the mirror today…and I thought I looked like something from outer space. I knew I would see myself like that. It's just a little bit too soon yet.
>
> (What do you see when you look in the mirror?)
>
> A ruined face, really….Half of it anyway, and it makes me feel very angry…very, very angry….I'd really like to get out of here and just get back into my life and forget what happened, and that's impossible….It's not as though I am going to walk out of here with a face that's exactly like what it was before. I can see that now. It's not going to be the same. There are going to be differences, and people are going to notice differences….I think that I will feel very, very vulnerable out in the open.
>
> The [left] hand has never been anything great for me to look at. I've never really been able to pick it up and lift it up and say, "Doesn't it look wonderful?" or "Isn't that looking better?" At the moment it's pretty horrible.
>
> (What does it feel like?)
>
> It feels like an old woman's hand, and it looks like about a 90-year-old woman's hand….It doesn't look like mine. I look at this [injured, left] hand here, and then I look at that one [uninjured, right]; they are not the same at all….In a funny sort of way I can't really see myself as myself again. Not really. I think I've got a long way to go before that happens.

Other patients with burn injuries described similar feelings of alienation and feelings of anger at not being able to escape their situation. Their injured bodies *would not* (and could not) *go away.* However strange and even grotesque their appearance, these *were* their own bodies, the only bodies through which they could be in the world.

For patients with cancer, *looking different* came on more gradually and occurred for a variety of reasons. Some patients who did not lose hair as the result of chemotherapy and maintained a steady body weight found it reassuring that they still looked (even if they did not feel) the same. Others were reassured, at least initially, that even though they looked different this was not necessarily apparent to others. The two women who had breast cancer, for example, both developed lymphoedema (a marked swelling of the arm and hand as a result of the accumulation of lymph [fluid] in the tissues), but by wearing long-sleeved clothing, they were largely able to conceal the swelling. Neither woman felt as successful in her later attempts to conceal the loss of hair that occurred half-way through the chemotherapy cycle.

Fears of *looking different* sometimes led to drastic, but ultimately ineffective actions, which only added to patients' discomfort. For example, in the attempt to prevent hair loss, which commonly occurs with some chemotherapeutic drugs, some patients were offered and, at least initially, accepted "the cold cap,"[2] an extremely uncomfortable and even painful procedure that offered no guarantee that hair loss would not occur. Once it became apparent, however, that even this drastic measure was not effective in a particular case, patients were relieved to be able to go through the procedure of having chemotherapy without the added discomfort and time involved in wearing the cold cap. Even though they felt the loss of hair very keenly and found wigs neither comfortable nor an adequate substitute for their own hair, there was a limit to what they felt able to endure in order to prevent the inevitable impact of chemotherapy.

Patients with burn injuries faced a sudden change in the way they looked, and they hoped that with healing and treatment they would regain some if not most of their previous appearance. Patients with cancer, on the other hand, started out looking normal and unchanged but experienced progressive changes in the way they looked to themselves and to others as the result of surgery, chemotherapy, and the progression of cancer.

Having cancer and receiving chemotherapy increasingly came to mean not only *looking different*, but also fearing the significance of the visible and felt changes in one's embodied self. Even as they felt dis-ease in how they looked to themselves and especially to others, patients with cancer also felt *trapped* in their particular bodies and in a web of uncertainties about the future. Like patients with burns, they, too, came to understand that their lives could be lived only through the ailing bodies from which they sometimes felt repulsed but could not escape. The following exemplar comes from a middle-aged man on his first cycle of intravenous chemotherapy, and he describes what it is like to have chronic leukemia:

> My feeling generally about it is that I've caught something. It's a virus thing that starts it apparently....It's done its damage, and I am stuck with this body and what is going on in it and is going to have to go on....I don't quite know the effect it has on glands, but it does seem as though your lymph system generally is overloaded with everything, and your glands, the good cells, are trying to do their bit, but there is too many of the others [diseased cells] for them to do their bit. So of course everything looks full....The thing that bothers me is how I look sometimes. My glands come up over here, under the chin, and that's fairly noticeable. They get really quite large. They are uncomfortable....I feel confused. Oh, I feel hopeless about it sometimes. I know I can't get away from it....I think it's a feeling of being trapped; you know you are trapped, but then, that's life.

The obvious changes in appearance brought about by injuries and scarring, by hair loss, or by changes in body weight were only one part of *looking different*. Because they felt different, patients also felt that others would be able to see the difference, and in a way they did. What others saw were often the subtle changes, changes that the patients themselves were not always fully aware: the loss of sparkle in the eye, the change in posture as the shoulders sagged, the hesitation in their step as they walked into the clinic or toward the treatment room. *Looking different* to others elicited responses from them, which in turn reinforced the patients' feelings that they not only *looked* different, but *were* different. Concerns about how people outside the hospital would respond to their *looking different* in turn added to the patients' feelings of vulnerability and a sense of isolation within their embodied selves.

Feeling different and being different

To have cancer or burn injuries is to *feel different* and to experience oneself as *being different*. For patients with burn injuries, the awareness that they were different came suddenly and forcefully. They talked of *the shock* of initial trauma and the realization that something was very wrong with their bodies, which they felt was no longer under their control. A woman who had spilled burning wax over her arm and chest provided a vivid description of being let down by her body, which would no longer respond in expected and habitual ways:

I just looked at my arm, and there was all this white skin...."Oh," I said, "that's bad." I sat down on the floor...because I felt weak. He [husband] was trying to get me to stand up, and I couldn't. I said, "My legs won't, I just can't"...and then I fainted.

Patients with burns also felt uncomfortable and restricted in their ability to move, *restrained* in a body that *felt different* and limited their range of options of being in the world. It was not only that they were confined to hospital or a particular room, but that their habitual postures and movements were no longer available to them. They felt restricted by bandages and dressings as well as by exposed burns oozing blood and serous exudate and tightening across wounds as the surface dried. The following exemplar captures the sense of being *caught in a situation* and *feeling trapped* within one's own body:

I am still restricted in bending my arms and turning my head and bending down. I don't go all the way because of burns and the blistering.

(Can you tell me what that feels like?)

Oh, you can imagine yourself being a fly in a cobweb, and you don't know where to move. You are just sticky, and you can't move anywhere, and your feet are glued down to the web. You can move, but you are restricted as to much movement. Not very much movement at all. You are getting nowhere....[The skin] feels very tight, very tight. And it all feels like it's dripping down on my face but at the same time stretching my face.

As their wounds healed and they became more comfortable and free in their movements, patients with burns started to regain some sense of their previous habitual bodies (discussed later in this chapter). They felt that the worst was behind them and that even if regaining a sense of wholeness was a slow process they were moving in the right direction.

For patients with cancer, the experience was rather different. For them, *feeling different* started with a gradual intimation of something being wrong and was intensified as they underwent diagnostic procedures and commenced chemotherapy. In the early stages, they *felt anxious* and *insecure* about what was going on inside their bodies, about the tests and investigations they had to undergo, and about the significance of having cancer and needing chemotherapy. In the midst of these concerns, they also had to gain a new understanding of their bodies and bodily sensations. For these patients, diagnostic procedures[3] meant being exposed to intrusive, unpleasant, and sometimes painful experiences and having to accept that such experiences would be repeated in the future. For those with little past experience of pain, the pain of diagnostic procedures was the first personally experienced indication that having cancer might mean having pain.

Having chemotherapy brought its own feelings of *being different* and being made different by the impact of *having to have chemotherapy* and the effects of particular drugs. Patients described the difficult situation of feeling better between treatments but not on the days following chemotherapy. The struggle for them was to submit to therapy that made them feel *uncomfortable, depressed,* and *different* when they knew that the ultimate benefits of chemotherapy were uncertain. Thus, patients with cancer also felt *trapped*, not in a situation of physical restriction, but in a situation in which they had no choice. To have chemotherapy was to accept others' decisions and to endure the consequences of those decisions, even as patients felt increasingly more uncertain about their ability to face the treatment and to endure it. Feeling depressed and helpless in the knowledge that *there is nothing I can do* exemplified patients' experience of having to have chemotherapy:

> When I am not having it [chemotherapy], I sort of feel quite good. And then, when I go to have one I think, "Oh, I don't know if I can handle having another one," but I know I have to go on, put up with it. Sometimes I get a little depressed, but I know that I just have to have it. There is nothing I can do.

Having chemotherapy also meant learning to live with a particular type of anxiety, *the dread*, that the treatment engendered. For the patients, the quantifiable aspects of the experience, such as the duration of the procedure or the degree of tissue damage entailed in its performance, were not the determining factors in the overall perception of the situation. However hard they tried to adopt a positive attitude, having chemotherapy meant having to live with its subjective *awfulness*. Because of its ability to act not only on the disease, but to change the whole person and the person's being in the world, chemotherapy inspired both awe and dread. As one patient expressed it,

> The dread of coming here. It's a bit like going to the dentist; the dread of it is probably worse than actually having it done....Just a general feeling of hating to come and hating to have it done and hating to have to have it done.

For some patients, *the dread* of chemotherapy extended beyond the clinic visits and the intravenous administration of drugs. For them, the disease and the drugs were imbued with powers that reduced the person to a helpless witness to a battle between the cancer that had taken over the body and the chemotherapy that aimed to destroy or at least control the disease. In such a situation, the person felt not only different, but *alienated from his/her own body* and unable to exert any significant control over his/her future. The once familiar body had become a battlefield:

> The cancer is either going to control me, or the medicine is going to control me, and apart from doing what I am told, and my diet, and things like that, I don't think that there is anything personally that I can do. Either the cancer is going to win, or the medicine is going to win. I don't know.

> (Where does that leave you?)

> It leaves me with a real horrible feeling in that I don't know which is going to win. I know which one I want!...It's either going to be the medicine or the cancer that wins, and there is not a lot I can do, I don't think.

Feeling different also meant *feeling that one had lost the taken-for-granted ease of being in the world* and having to live with tiredness, depression, and cyclical highs and lows in terms of mood and energy. Patients generally expected chemotherapy to be more painful and more obviously unpleasant while it was being administered but that otherwise they would feel normal. In fact, what they experienced was frequently more insidious and difficult to understand and communicate to others. As the following exemplar shows, many seemingly minor changes and sensations had a cumulative effect on the person who felt different and *not herself*, not only during the treatment, but also in the days following it:

> I felt a little drowsy after the first treatment [anti-emetic drug] had gone through, and I was just feeling that it would be nice when it was finished...when all the little vials had gone through....It's not a painful thing. It's almost a suffocating feeling that is swamping you, I guess. It is going through your system, and I would just like it to be over and done with....I do feel this sort of suffocating type of feeling. I am not in control of my body, and I am having drugs put into my body, and therefore I just feel out of control.

There was a tiredness when I finished the treatment. I went home and took it fairly easily and just tried to relax....The only other effect I noticed was the mouth, there was a dryness and a strange feeling on the tongue. The throat seemed to be a little enlarged; the actual glands felt enlarged. This feeling wore off after about two days....I wasn't quite sure how the body would react, and I thought it had reacted very well.

I found that I felt a little odd in the stomach...and I just generally felt a little seedy....You generally felt that you were getting around with a bit of a seedy body, but you weren't actually sick. You wouldn't go and lie down and take to bed like you were ill, but you just weren't...quite yourself.

It had a depressing angle about it that I hadn't expected. I felt very depressed taking the treatment, and the rest of the day and perhaps the next day I felt in quite a state of depression about it, I don't really know why.

The absence of disease-related pain in patients with cancer, either as a presenting symptom or during the period of the study, contrasted with the almost constant presence of pain for patients with burns. The latter were made different not only by the wounds and eventual scars that altered their appearance, they were also made different by their experiences of *pain*, which signalled the initial trauma and which, to a lesser or greater degree, persisted throughout their time of hospitalization and treatment. Patients' expectations that their pain would be relieved once they arrived at the hospital and received professional care were often not fulfilled. As a result, they had to learn to endure not only the painful procedures of saline baths, wound debridement and dressing changes, but also the background wound pain that was present at other times and the residual pain that often persisted for half an hour or longer following the completion of particularly painful procedures involving burn wounds.

The persistence and further infliction of pain increased patients' feelings of vulnerability and diminished their hopes of ever being as they were before the accident. Initial injuries and subsequent treatments changed their being-in-the-world, and everything around them seemed not only different, but also out of their control. As one young man expressed it,

Still sore. There is always pain....I can't sleep at night, so a lot of things have changed. My sleeping habits, my eating habits. It's just sort of...I've come into a whole new world....It makes the time go slow. See, I want the time to go fast, but I am trying too hard to make it go fast.

Whether in hospital recovering from burn injuries or at home and attending the out-patient clinic for chemotherapy, patients in the study felt different and profoundly changed by their situation. They experienced themselves as inhabiting bodies that felt strange and unpredictable, bodies that made them uncomfortable and uneasy. Their previous feelings of being out-in-the-world and able to shape the world around them were replaced, at least for a time, with feelings of being disconnected from the world and trapped in bodies that restricted their actions and their choices. In this context, having chemotherapy or treatment for burn injuries meant enduring that which they hoped would return them to their previous feeling of being themselves. However unpleasant, uncomfortable or painful, treatment held a promise, a hope of recovery of the former self. There were experiences during this time, however, that patients felt threatened to overwhelm them and made them poignantly aware of the fragility of their existence and the limits to their capacity to endure.

Feeling overwhelmed

For patients in the study, being burned involved very strong feelings of fear: of what their bodies looked like, that the pain would not stop and that they may not survive the injuries and the pain. It involved feelings of confusion about the specific circumstances surrounding the accident, the extent of their injuries, and the meaning of sensations of extreme cold, burning, and pain. The suddenness and intensity of initial pain was so overpowering for some patients that they felt unable to stop crying or screaming. Reassurances from emergency and hospital staff that they were safe and would recover seemed meaningless and unrelated to their personal situation. They felt *frightened, helpless,* and *vulnerable,* not only in the immediate situation, but also later, especially when severe pain returned during painful procedures. To experience burn injuries was to know *the immediacy of severe pain* as an extreme experience that floods the person's consciousness and makes it difficult to attend to anything else but the pain and one's profound need for relief from it. The following two exemplars capture *the feeling of being overwhelmed by pain.* For a young woman in this study, the initial experience of pain was so overpowering that she evaluated all her subsequent encounters with pain in the light of this experience:

The first pain I felt was my face, my hand, and then it was all over [the body] and it was just steady...steady is not the right word. It was just the most incredible pain. I really can't find the words for it....I cried all the time....I was busy wondering if the pain was actually going to go....I thought that the feeling was just permanent....[Even after reaching hospital and being given Morphine intravenously, her pain did not diminish.]...It was so painful then. It was just as painful. Probably part of that was the shock, but more than anything it was just the actual pain. It was pain that I would not like to inflict on anybody.

When it first happened, it went on for a *long, long time*. I will never forget that total burning, that *body burning*. It just felt like my whole body was burning. I can remember...it wasn't one particular area that I could isolate. My whole body was burning, and it was almost like an uncontrollable pain....Uncontrollable, absolutely nothing anybody could do.

At the same time as medical assessment confirmed "15 percent burns," this woman's lived experience was not of discrete areas of injury but of her whole body hurting and losing its intactness. To suffer such severe trauma was *to lose a sense of one's bodily boundaries* and to be overwhelmed by pain. To suffer extensive burns and prolonged, severe pain was also *to doubt one's will to live* and to fear for one's very survival. In the next quote, the young man expresses his feelings of vulnerability and fear but also of a determination to fight back:

A lot of the time I am scared. When it first happened I was scared I was never going to live. 'Cause I just didn't think I had the will power to get through it myself, because the pain was far too much then....When I first went in [to hospital] I didn't think I was going to make it....I am scared that when the pain increases too much, I am scared that I might just give in and not be able to pull through....I've got to fight this pain. Just to prove that I can beat it, then I know I'll get better.

For patients with cancer, *feeling overwhelmed* was not related to pain, although, to some degree, fear of pain was usually a factor in the situation. Having undergone a number of painful diagnostic procedures and faced with chemotherapy, which they knew to be potent, patients feared how their individual bodies would react to this treatment and how they would cope with it. The fear of what chemotherapy might do to them and what they were allowing others to do to their bodies made the first chemotherapy treatment into an experience charged with anxiety and fear. For some patients the anxiety was overwhelming, as in the following interview excerpt where the patient describes his extreme apprehension and, in the same interview, his reaction to the first session of chemotherapy:

> Within myself I was very anxious beforehand. I didn't know what to expect. Oh, I knew it was an injection, but I was very, very anxious beforehand. I didn't know what kind of reaction I was going to have. I had this stupid dream last night, where I had a seizure.

(Tell me about that.)

> Oh, it was weird. I was lying on the bed, with nurse on one side and doctor on the other, and for some reason, they gave me this injection, but it was in my foot of all places. I could see it there, in my foot. And as soon as the injection went in…this weird feeling came over me. A throbbing, shaking, you know. I was trying to say to this nurse, "Help me, help me!" but there was nothing coming out. Although I knew I was saying it, they could not hear me. I just woke up, I think, and it had gone, but it was so vivid that it made me feel really apprehensive.

> Actual sitting down here, it's like sitting in an electric chair. They do all this preparation and then you have it. And then this sudden flood or wave came over me and I felt bad. I felt really bad…light headed, dizzy, as if I was going to pass out.…I am still apprehensive about what sort of reaction I am going to have. Whether I am going to be sick later in the day, or whether I am going to feel faint.

Feeling overwhelmed was a profoundly disturbing experience that both groups of patients found difficult to share with others. It was as though they were on the edge of an abyss with nothing to hang on to. Feeling overwhelmed by pain or anxiety placed the patients in a situation of utter helplessness where not only the world, but their own bodies had lost their previously known and predictable realities. Instead, both had become hostile and uncomfortable. It was difficult for patients to talk about such experiences, not only because words were difficult to find, but also because they could not do so without crying and exposing their vulnerability. Some patients found it difficult to open themselves up to their families, either because to do so would have been out of character or because questions that would have prompted the patient to talk about the experience of feeling overwhelmed were not asked. Research interviews provided opportunities for some to relate their experiences and express their feelings. One patient who cried during three of the four interviews conducted with him commented that being able to cry had helped him to come to terms with what had happened to him:

> I needed prompting, like your questions, to get me started. Then I can talk about how it *really* feels.

Talking about their experience, including the traumatic aspects of that experience, was one way in which patients were able to move toward the recovery of their former selves. They needed to regain a sense of wholeness and a sense of ease in their embodied being, yet many of the treatment procedures they had to undergo reinforced their feelings of being different and of not having control over their bodies and their lives. To *feel myself again*, to regain a sense of personal embodiment, was a common desire for patients with cancer as well as those with burn injuries. While some endured the treatments and the set-backs with hope, others found it difficult to believe that they would ever feel whole again.

REGAINING THE HABITUAL BODY AND BECOMING ONESELF AGAIN

For the patients in the study, being ill or injured involved a loss of their previously known and familiar selves. For some this was a temporary loss, which they were able to overcome, albeit with some effort. For others it was a devastating experience from which they could see no way out. They felt trapped and powerless in a situation that they felt unable to alter. For patients with cancer, *becoming oneself again* happened at two levels: first, following each round of chemotherapy and, second, as a long-term process of accepting their changed situation and going on living. To a certain extent *becoming oneself again* and *regaining one's habitual body* just happened, especially to patients with burns. As their wounds healed and the pain diminished, as they were able to walk around and sleep through the night, and as others commented on their improving appearance, so these patients talked of *starting to feel my old self again*. And yet regaining a sense of one's former self was not something that merely happened. Through their experiences of illness and injury, patients were able to reevaluate their past views and actions and, in some cases, make plans for a different future.

Becoming oneself again required that patients see themselves moving toward a better future rather than remaining trapped in their present or wishing for a magical return to a happier past. Some patients arrived at a point where they were able to see themselves as themselves again; others struggled to do so but were only partly successful; while still others experienced the distress of feeling trapped and alienated within permanently marred bodies. Whether achieved or not, for the patients in this study, *becoming oneself again* meant being able to leave behind feelings of dis-ease, vulnerability, fear and uncertainty; feelings of being trapped, helpless and powerless; and sometimes feelings of anger and resentment. *Regaining one's habitual body* and *becoming oneself again* also meant regaining a sense of bodily intactness, feeling safe from harm, being in control of one's emotions, and being able to make decisions that mattered. Being oneself again meant feeling that one is a whole being, back in the mainstream of life, connected to the world—the scars and the possible future treatments notwithstanding. There were several ways in which patients were able to achieve a sense of being oneself again. These different ways involved different patterns of seeing oneself and being in the world.

Resuming the interrupted flow of life

For one group of patients, all with burn injuries, achieving a sense of *being oneself again* appeared almost effortless. It was an integral part of the healing process. The injuries were an unwelcome interruption in the flow of an otherwise secure life. Their bodies were injured, and they suffered as the result of pain and as the result of losing their habitual, taken-for-granted sense of embodiment. Despite this, however, they did not doubt that they would recover, that they would resume their previous home and job responsibilities, or that people who mattered in their life would be supportive and understanding. Even when they could not take their bodies for granted or endure the pain with as much stoicism and composure as they wished, they felt able to count on others, particularly their families. Their sense of who they were and where they belonged was not challenged by the experience of injury and hospitalization. They took pleasure in every sign of healing and welcomed the treatments and the ministrations of others as a necessary part of regaining their sense of embodiment and becoming themselves again:

> I felt glad that she was cutting it [debriding dead skin] off, and I could see the smooth skin again underneath....I suppose it's a good feeling to know that underneath the dead skin there is life again; there is new skin again underneath.

> You are reliant upon someone else to do what they can for you.

(How does that feel?)

I don't know how to answer that...but I know it wasn't me, it wasn't my body. I felt as if I was getting help from other people to give me back what was mine before all this [burn injuries] happened. I suppose your body has been through a big shock. Your body has to readjust....I was glad for the physio[therapist] coming in to give me back movement in my fingers to start off with. It was really quite sore while she worked on it. And then she worked on my wrist and I felt "oh, good, something's coming back." And she actually got on to my elbow, and I felt "hurrah, I've got my arm back!" You do feel as if you've lost part of your body, and you rely on others to give it back to you.

Creating a new kind of future

For two patients, the impact of what had happened to them was much more than a temporary interruption. Their life could not resume where it had left off a few weeks previously. There was no longer a settled pattern of life to which they could return. The only way they could proceed into the future was as changed persons, with new knowledge and a fresh outlook. Having cancer and receiving chemotherapy and surviving extensive burn injuries constituted a crisis, a turning point beyond which life had to be lived differently. Both patients lacked close family support and felt that they had gone through the trauma of their experience alone. Yet the trauma was worthwhile since it offered the possibility of a new life.

For the patient who accepted that her advanced breast cancer could only be held at bay with chemotherapy, becoming herself again involved accepting the trauma of chemotherapy in exchange for the hope of a future. At the age of 46, she no longer expected her *three score years and ten*, but neither did she give up on life. She prepared to take a long-planned trip abroad with a friend, to gradually resume her gardening and social activities and, when she felt strong enough, to return to work she had given up half-way through the chemotherapy program. In the meantime, she took slow walks by the sea, saw friends, and rested. Reflecting on 3 months of chemotherapy, she acknowledged both the trauma of the experience and her awareness of a worthwhile future:

It's a traumatic experience because it's an experience that, no matter how kind people are, you go through it on your own. There is only yourself that can go through it and handle it, and I don't think perhaps other people understand quite how you feel about it.

I did feel there was some hope [in accepting chemotherapy].…I feel I've got a future, and for however long it is, I am going to make the best of it. That's why I am persevering with having the treatment that they want me to have because I am sure it will be of help to me.

The patient who knew that he had nearly died in a house fire later experienced such severe pain that he thought he might not be able to endure it and might die. For a person who had been physically abused as a child, who used violence to assert his claims and settle disagreements with friends and enemies alike, to feel helpless and afraid in the face of so much pain was a new and deeply disturbing experience. He could not hit back but had to endure the pain. For the first time in his life, he was able to appreciate how helpless and defenseless his girlfriend would have felt when confronted by his violent behavior and why she had left him, taking their young child with her. His suffering forced him to reassess his values and the impact of his actions on those who were estranged by his violent behavior. In a sense, his pain and suffering had constituted him into a person, with a new understanding of his past and plans for a different future. For this young man, *becoming himself again* involved becoming a person who liked himself and his changed outlook, despite the physical scars, and who hoped that others would like him better as the result. It was a painful experience of self-discovery, but it was an experience that gave him hope for the future.

Fighting to remain a person

For some patients, *becoming oneself again* involved a continuing struggle against becoming totally passive and powerless observers of their wounded bodies. They felt able to endure the pain and the discomforts of their illness and injuries but not the passive acquiescence frequently demanded of them. They wanted to be consulted, informed, and involved in decisions about their treatments. They were keen observers of their condition and the effects different techniques and drugs had on them. They questioned others' actions, even when they knew that such questioning would make them unpopular with staff. Above all, they needed to be active participants in their therapy, to do their share and not simply trust that what others were doing was all that was necessary. A patient with burns, for example, asked for analgesic drugs he felt were more effective than those offered by particular nurses. He summoned his family to visit him when he felt in need of their support, and he obtained permission for his wife to assist with his baths until his facial swelling had subsided and he was able to see again.

For a patient with cancer, each cycle of chemotherapy was a struggle as she felt threatened by its effects on her. The normal pattern of her daily activities was disrupted by nausea, tiredness and feelings of depression following each new round of intravenous drugs. During the week when she took Prednisone™ she slept little, took up jogging, and did hours of gardening in addition to her other work. When this drug was withdrawn, she felt tired and listless and unable to accomplish even basic household chores. She felt that her body was controlled by drugs she had to accept and that she would *regain her habitual body* and *become herself again* only by asserting herself through her own choices and actions. As the following excerpt illustrates, for this patient, adhering to a particular diet was part of her fight to remain an active person, making choices and acting on them:

> I am eating a hundred percent raw [vegetarian] diet at the moment, and I really feel good in myself. Whether it does me any good or not, I feel good because *I am doing something for myself.* Something that I feel is going to be helpful.

> That's the big thing, the thought that I am doing something for myself. I don't want to just sit back and let people be doing things to me….I want to get better, and there's things I want to do. I want to go back to work and get some money, take trips overseas. So I'd rather aim for that, and I know it mightn't work out that way, but at least I am trying, and it makes me feel so much better, the knowing that I am trying.

Patients who were able to regain a sense of being themselves again had a particular perspective of their treatments and the associated pain and discomforts. They accepted them as necessary and bearable but did not see them as the only means through which their bodies would heal. An important part of being able to become oneself again was their ability to draw on others' support, on their own inner resources, and to take action on their own behalf. Others, however, struggled and were only partly successful in feeling that they were becoming themselves again.

Living through each round of treatment

For some patients, having cancer and going through a lengthy period of chemotherapy was so destructive to their former selves that all they could do was to try and live through each round of treatment. One patient was sure that *God would heal her eventually*, but that in the meantime, she had to *walk through the deepest valley* and accept her suffering. Another patient was much less certain of her future, and in reordering her life (giving up paid work, attending daily mass, and doing charitable work), she seemed as concerned with death as with life. For both of these patients, each round of chemotherapy was something to be endured, a trial that became more difficult to face as the treatment progressed. Their concern was to regain a sense of being themselves again after each session of chemotherapy, but in the meantime, their life was in limbo. They felt unable to talk about their experience of illness and chemotherapy with family and friends, tried to hide their distress from others, and tried not to think of it too much themselves. For them, *becoming oneself again* meant feeling the worst effects of chemotherapy subsiding and being able to resume their daily activities a day at a time. They felt that their lives were ruled by chemotherapy and that they could not exert any influence over the situation they were in other than living through each round of treatment. *Being oneself* was a temporary achievement that lasted only until the next treatment round approached:

> I psyche myself up a day or so before I actually find I am coming in. Talk myself into it generally, "That's where I am going and that's what I am going to do."…It's difficult to take things in your stride and just treat it as a normal occurrence. With everyday activities, you don't psyche yourself up for them. They just happen. This is quite a major thing. You are coming along for treatment, and you definitely have to get into a state of mind for it.

> When the treatment started and the needle was being put in, I felt…I'd lost control.

> I think it's just the thought of drugs invading your body and the power of the drugs. They are setting up reactions, and there is a slightly depressing effect with them, too. I think this is why you feel you are not yourself until you've slept and started your next day without the thought that you are going to have these drugs.

Living with persistent feeling of not being oneself

Finally, there were patients who felt so changed by their experience that, at least for the time being, they could not see themselves as themselves again. They felt alienated and even repulsed by their bodies and talked about them as *uncooperative* (when they would *not behave themselves* and yield blood specimens easily) or as *hostile* entities (that interfered with their rest and sleep). They felt *let down* by bodies that could no longer be relied on to look and feel normal, and they felt trapped in bodies and situations that they wished to leave but realized they could not. Feeling strange and not oneself was particularly disturbing in the early stages of chemotherapy, as vividly captured by a patient's description of his reactions to his first round of chemotherapy:

> A bit strange….It was a funny kind of feeling. Almost as if I was beside myself. As if it was really sort of me looking on….I went home and didn't feel sick…I went home and slept. But it was really strange. I've had some weird, funny feelings this week. Whether it's the medication, the tablets, and everything else, or whether it's just me, I am not sure….Dizzy as if…dizzy, as if it's not me. I don't seem to have any control over myself. I can't breathe and I am hot. Real dizzy. My eyes tend to go out of focus….I don't seem to be able to control what I am doing.

Feeling overwhelmed by what was happening to them, the two patients with cancer tended to dwell on the limitations of their treatment and the chances that either it would be ineffective in their case from the beginning or that eventually it would no longer work. Each round of treatment was thus a potent reminder of their illness and their dependence on chemotherapy and their precarious hold on life. Within this context, they felt vulnerable, out of control, and trapped within strange bodies and an uncertain future.

A persistent feeling of not being oneself was not limited to patients with cancer. For a patient who had suffered extensive burns, regaining a sense of embodiment and wholeness seemed an impossible task. She acknowledged that some of her wounds had healed well and knew that she would have further plastic surgery over the following year to achieve better cosmetic results. As an embodied person, however, she still felt overwhelmed by the destructiveness of her injuries, and she could not see herself as a whole person again:

> I feel like I am made up of patches, and it's hard to know where the real me is under all these dressings and bandages.

> It didn't matter how many times I was told, it still didn't really mean…I wouldn't allow it to mean anything because I almost didn't

really believe it. Couldn't believe it. Couldn't find a little space in my mind there to believe [that she would heal and be herself again].

Feeling a need to *regain one's habitual body* and to be oneself again was an important part of the patients' experience of cancer and chemotherapy and burn injuries and treatment. It was a way of recognizing a need for a future, a need to see themselves not just as they had been, but as they would be beyond the period when they had to accept a loss of wholeness and their former selves. For some, becoming oneself again was almost like a gift that they embraced as they returned to the flow of their everyday life. For others, it was a struggle not to be lost in total dependence on others and to assert their right to be active participants in the healing process. For some, it was a chance to discover a new sense of self and to create a different kind of personal future. For others, the present proved too overwhelming, and becoming oneself again was too distant a possibility, which they felt was beyond their grasp.

It was in this context of changed embodiment and a struggle to regain a sense of their familiar selves that patients experienced a series of diagnostic and treatment procedures that were often uncomfortable, painful, and sometimes distressing. Their desire for healing and for a future in which they could be themselves again helped them to look at the procedures as necessary and at nurses' actions in performing the procedures as legitimate. Nevertheless, enduring discomfort and pain associated with such procedures added to their feelings of being changed and of being vulnerable, exposed and lacking control over themselves and over their world. It is within this context of changed embodiment and changed being-in-the-world that the phenomenon of inflicted pain is explored and described in the following chapters.

ENDNOTES

[1]This occurred frequently since the Oncology Clinic rooms had no windows and patients had only bare walls to look at during treatments. The treatment room in the Burn Care Unit had large windows with pleasant views, but patients sometimes had to be treated in their beds, with curtains pulled around for privacy, when the treatment room was needed for another patient.

[2]A tight fitting, helmet-like cap made of thick, soft fabric. The cap is soaked in water, placed over a skull-shaped mould, and placed in a freezer for several hours. Prior to the administration of intravenous chemotherapy, the patient's hair is moist-

ened with cold water and the frozen cap is fitted over the head. To achieve its aim of reducing the likelihood of hair loss, the cap has to be worn for at least 10 minutes before the commencement of chemotherapy, as well as during treatment, and for 20 minutes after its completion.

[3]All patients with cancer who participated in the study underwent at least three of the following investigative (and intrusive) procedures: venepunctures; needle biopsies; radiographic investigations such as mammography, arteriography, or lymphangiography; computerized scans; bone marrow aspirations, and more extensive surgical procedures such as laparotomies needed to establish the presence of primary or secondary tumors and to obtain biopsies.

Chapter 4
The Phenomenon of Clinically Inflicted Pain: Essential Themes

In writing about the essential qualities of bodily pain, Scarry (1985) makes the point that we experience pain in such a way that it is simultaneously "something that cannot be denied and something that cannot be confirmed" (p. 13). In other words, "to have pain is to have *certainty*; to hear about pain is to have *doubt*." In this chapter, my aim is to describe the lived experience of people who came to know the certainty of pain, in particular, inflicted pain.

Rather than merely recording individual experiences, this chapter deals with the *essential themes* of the experience of inflicted pain, themes that address the qualities of the phenomenon without which it would not be what it is (van Manen, 1990, p. 107). Through the processes of data analysis and interpretation, as well as ongoing reflection, four key themes emerged and best capture the essential qualities of the phenomenon of clinically inflicted pain: *the hurt and the painfulness of inflicted pain; handing one's body over to others; expectation and experience of being wounded;* and *restraining the body and the voice.*

The implied assumption of much existing research is that clinically inflicted pain is no different from other types of acute pain. In setting aside this assumption, my aim has been to turn to the lived experience of those with direct knowledge of inflicted pain and to be open to whatever their experiences may reveal about the phenomenon. What the study has identified is that inflicted pain is both like other pain and at the same time unlike any other pain. The blending of these common and unique qualities is what constitutes the particular phenomenon of inflicted pain. The four essential themes are used to structure the description of the phenomenon, while exemplars help to "maintain a strong and oriented relation" (van Manen, 1990, p. 135), a constant connection to the lifeworld of particular individuals whose experiences have made the understanding of the phenomenon possible.

Themes that relate to how patients perceive those who inflict pain on them, how they are affected by the experience of inflicted pain, and how they interpret and give meaning to the experience are presented in the next chapter. While these additional themes may be termed *incidental* (van Manen, 1990, p. 106) since they only indirectly address the nature of the phenomenon of inflicted pain, they are nevertheless vitally important in the project of contextual understanding that this study aims to achieve.

THE HURT AND THE PAINFULNESS OF INFLICTED PAIN

The essential quality of inflicted pain, like other pain, is that it *hurts*. It is *painful*. It is itself, and it is itself only when experienced as an abnormal but integral quality of embodied existence. Pain imposes its presence by its intensity as well as by its spatiality, its particular location within the body. Without an outside point of reference, pain resists objectification, and its essential qualities of hurt and painfulness are difficult to express in language and thus difficult to share with others. Whatever others may understand about a person's pain, its essential painfulness can only be lived, not shared. This perhaps is why even the most articulate and communicative of patients often prefaced descriptions of their experiences with statements about their inability to put their experience into words. It is not that their accounts lacked vividness, urgency, or evocative power, but that they knew that there was more to their experience than even the most eloquent speech could convey.

For the patients with burn injuries, the *sheer painfulness*, *immediacy*, and *inescapable bodily presence* of inflicted pain meant that such pain became the central concern of their experience of treatment. Some concerns, such as those related to job, household or financial responsibilities, were often taken over by others, and patients were encouraged to allow others to "worry about" such matters. To some extent even concerns about current disfigurement and eventual scarring were able to be postponed until grafting surgery had taken place and dressings were taken off. In the first few days, patients were either unable to see their wounds or chose not to look at them during dressing changes. Severe bodily pain, however, could not be denied, postponed, or handed over to someone else for a time. It had to be lived through and endured. The condition of the person's continued conscious embodiment was the consciousness of pain.

In the context of burn trauma, diagnostic and treatment procedures were performed on patients already in pain. Pain for them was not just something that happened on isolated occasions, even though it did become more intense at particular times. Their experience was of severe, even overwhelming pain, of pain that affected their whole being, sapped their energies, challenged their views of themselves and cast doubt on their recovery. Pain exerted a constant presence that came to represent the experience of burn trauma and recovery. In the stark words of one patient,

> I have never experienced quite as much pain. *Never ever* had so much pain [as in the previous four weeks].

So much pain could refer to either the intensity of pain or to its persistence, but it usually meant both. Patients quite often felt overwhelmed by the nature and severity of the pain, the duration of the painful procedures, and their own inability to anticipate accurately where and how much pain they would experience. Their familiar being-in-the-world was changed into unpredictable and often painful encounters with the world, which had become hostile. One of the early experiences for patients was the realization that even the most taken-for-granted prerequisites for life, air and water, could be the instruments of pain. In the first exemplar, the patient is describing his experience of having dressings removed from his burned legs and hands and waiting a few minutes to be lowered into a bath:

> As soon as the wound is exposed to the air, I get very cold, and it actually makes them burn. The burns get cold, and then they feel like they burn....I don't know how to describe it, but it doesn't quite get to the unbearable stage. But it is awfully sore, pretty sore.

In the second exemplar, a patient who prided himself on his ability to withstand pain in other contexts describes the shock of realizing how painful having his first saline bath was for him. What this exemplar also captures is the patient's awareness that this same pain, which has left such a mark on him, is *unbelievable*. It is something about which he is very certain, and yet, if it had not happened to him, he, too, would have found it difficult to believe that pain could hurt as much:

> It's hard to express what the pain is like…you would have to experience it to understand it, and I don't think I would ever want to experience it again.…I would put it close to a 10, between 8 and 10 [on a 10-point scale].…The sensations were unreal. It was just unbelievable.…When my back was uncovered, it was just unbelievable. Even the cold air was enough to make you scream.…That was the first time I have ever known water to hurt a person. It's like salt. It was like salt going into a cut. Very painful.

Further pain related to specific nursing actions was often added to the pain arising from the wound's exposure to air or immersion in water. Actions such as the removal of dressings (and how this was done), leaving the wounds exposed, covering them with heavy and stiff cloth that stuck to the raw wound, and deliberately or inadvertently delaying the application of new dressings often increased patients' pain.

Unintended delays occurred when nurses had to attend to other patients or were called away to assist another nurse. Deliberate delays in applying new dressings occurred when wounds were to be inspected by the surgeons during medical rounds or when the nurses decided that the healing process would be aided by exposing wounds to air and allowing them to dry. Whatever the reasons, patients found that exposed wounds *hurt* as a burning sensation intensified and *tightened* as a thin, dry membrane formed across exposed raw tissues, *pulling* and causing increasing pain. Not understanding the rationale behind nurses' actions and not being given an explanation or even a warning that there would be pain made the experience particularly distressing for patients. The painfulness of the experience and the added distress of not knowing why it was necessary are captured in the following exemplar from two interviews with a patient who had suffered deep and extensive burns to most of the lateral aspect of her left arm in addition to less extensive burns to her chest and back. In the first incident, her wounds had been left exposed for over three hours; in the second incident, the wound was exposed for a slightly shorter period:

> I was all right for a start, but after a while the pain just started to get worse, so that I had to grip the side of the bed just to stop [shaking] and grit my teeth to cope with the pain. [I had to] keep that going all the time, and the pain just seemed to be there all the time.…It seemed to me to really hurt…my arm was the one that was hurting a lot.

The whole arm was squeezing together...pulling, tightening, all along my arm. It was exposed, and having a look at it seems to me I should see it pulling tighter and tighter....If it was explained to me, the reasons why they do that [leave burns exposed] I would have felt all right. I would have been prepared for it. But I wasn't! I almost burst into tears.

[Eventually, when alone] I did have a real good cry, sobbed my heart out.

An especially difficult type of pain for patients to cope with was the sudden, very intense *jolt of pain* that occurred in the middle of an already painful procedure, when a nurse touched a particularly sensitive spot such as an exposed nerve or tendon. The sheer intensity of such pain made patients feel totally defenseless and thereafter afraid of a repeat occurrence of similarly overwhelming pain. They hoped it would never be as painful as it had been, but they could never be sure that it would not be. Even the memory of such intense pain could reduce a patient to tears, as in the following exemplar from an interview with a middle-aged patient who never cried as an adult and could not remember crying even as a child:

They were cleaning off my hands, and they had cleaned my face off first using some solution, I am not sure what it was called. And then they proceeded to do my hands. But there was apparently some other solution on one of the nurse's gloves, just a trace of it. And when she touched my hand with it, that was worse than the original [pain, at the time of injury]. I couldn't stand it.

[Patient broke into loud sobs at this point. The interview was stopped and resumed some minutes later when patient indicated that he wished to continue.]

But that was exactly what happened. Like your hand held in the fire. So on your 1 to 10 scale it was 99, or 9.99. I can't think of anything worse, but there's got to be something. There is always something worse....It was probably 5 or 6 minutes, and that was equivalent of 5 or 6 days as far as I was concerned. It was that sore.

Something of the *hurt* and *painfulness* of inflicted pain may be discerned from the specific words used by patients with burns to describe the pain they experienced. Feelings of discomfort and low levels of unpleasant sensation were acknowledged and talked about but seldom described as pain. What qualified as pain for these patients was the experience that embodied both a sensory awareness of wounding (discussed in a later section) and a strong sense of its impact on them as whole persons. The terms listed in Table 4.1 give some indication of the severity of the sensory experience of pain as well as its impact on the person. When using such words patients often added emphasis by the tone of their voice or by the addition of qualifying terms terms such as *very* sore or *really* bad. (Note: The list follows that used in the McGill Pain Questionnaire [Melzack, 1975], but it includes additional terms used by the study participants.)

Sensory	Evaluative	Affective
burning	awful	crying
stinging	bad	frightening
searing	endless	distressing
sharp	horrible	tiring
sore	excruciating	exhausting
hurting	powerful	revolting
tender	unbearable	
pinching	overwhelming	
	extreme	

Table 4.1 Descriptive terms related to inflicted pain used by patients with burns

Decontextualized words and phrases are limited in their ability to convey the essential nature of inflicted pain. The essence of the lived experience of inflicted pain is that another's actions are not only hurting *my* leg or *my* back, a part of *my* body, *they are hurting me*. This is how patients experienced episodes of inflicted pain, and this experience is reflected in their descriptions. While some accounts included comments about the sensory qualities of pain, patients' descriptions tended to emphasize the affective and the evaluative qualities of the experience and its impact on them as persons. Thus, an episode of pain would be described not only as a *burning* or *searing* sensation, but also as something *awful, distressing,* or *overwhelming* in its impact on the person. The hurt and the painfulness of inflicted pain included its sensory qualities and the intensity dimension. But much more than that, it included its capacity to distress, frighten, and exhaust the patient and to challenge the patient's powers of endurance.

Unlike patients with burns, for whom inflicted pain came on top of considerable background pain stemming from the original injuries, patients with cancer who participated in the study did not experience pain either as a presenting symptom of their disease or as part of disease progression. For this group of patients, pain was confined to diagnostic and treatment procedures and occurred intermittently and for short periods of time. Despite being less frequent, of shorter duration, and involving less tissue damage than pain inflicted in the course of the treatment of burn injuries, pain associated with chemotherapy still had the essential qualities of hurting and painfulness. At times a procedure was performed without pain, but when there was pain, then it was real pain and not just something that "will not hurt" or "may only sting a little," as nurses frequently remarked prior to venepunctures. As one patient expressed it,

> Some days I don't feel it at all, and other days it really hurts....I suppose it really depends on whether they get the vein all right or not. If they get it all right, then it's OK, they can just sort of slip it in. The last one I had was really painful. I don't think I'd ever had it that bad before. It was quite sore.

Patients' inability to predict which procedures would be painful and how long they and the associated pain would last contributed to feelings of anxiety and apprehension prior to all procedures. Knowing that there was always the likelihood of pain and the unpleasant aftereffects associated with chemotherapy meant that patients had to summon courage to go through each clinic visit. Familiarity with regularly performed procedures such as venepunctures for purposes of obtaining blood samples or administering intravenous chemotherapy did not necessarily make these procedures either less painful or easier to tolerate. Having one's body invaded by instruments and drugs was experienced as *traumatic* and increasingly more difficult to tolerate as treatment progressed. Reflecting on 3 months of chemotherapy, the patient in the following exemplar captures the impact of repeated exposure to invasive procedures and chemotherapy on her:

> Very traumatic, that's how I feel it has affected me more than anything else....I have had to really build myself up for each session, then wind myself down again. It's a traumatic experience because it's an experience that, no matter how kind people are, you go through it on your own. There is only yourself that can go through it and handle it, and I don't think perhaps other people understand quite how you feel about it....To me, there was a lot of stress with going through it.

I was finding it worse as we got closer to the end....It doesn't get easier. And on reflection...I think it got harder.

In retrospect, patients considered painless venepunctures to have been a bonus rather than something they could expect with any confidence. As a result of local inflammatory changes and increasing fragility of veins used for chemotherapy administration, the incidence of unsuccessful venepunctures increased as the patient's treatment progressed. Instead of a single venepuncture in the diagnostic laboratory, followed by a single venepuncture in the Oncology Clinic, it was not uncommon for patients to have to endure two, three, or even more attempts to obtain a blood sample or insert a needle for chemotherapy administration. As this happened, the margin between tolerable and intolerable levels of pain narrowed, and the patients' sense of vulnerability increased. As the following exemplar shows, a single venepuncture may be acceptable, but repeated attempts could be quite distressing:

The worst time I've ever had was up on the wards. I came in because I had an infection, and they gave me an antibiotic drug. The young woman doctor had four goes and couldn't get it in, so she had to call someone else in. That was horrible, to keep going from one vein to the other and not being able to find it. I didn't like that. But when they find it the first time, it's fine.

Unlike patients with burns, for whom pain came to exemplify the experience of injury and recovery, patients with cancer had less frequent and less prolonged experiences of pain. Nevertheless, when present, inflicted pain (like any other pain) hurts, and while it lasts, it has to be endured. In terms of its hurt and painfulness then, inflicted pain is like other pain. What makes inflicted pain different from pathological pain resulting from a disease process is the need to allow another person to act on the patient's body, even when such actions cause pain. The fact that the patient allows others to act on his or her body also means that at least some of the patient's personal control has to be ceded to others. What is given over in such a situation, however, is not just a degree of control. What patients in the study described was the fact of handing over their own bodies to others to work on, even when such work entailed the infliction of pain.

HANDING ONE'S BODY OVER TO OTHERS

Pathological pain, arising out of physiological or pathological processes within the body, comes unbidden. The patient has no say in when such pain might start, how long it might last, or when it might return. In other words, people are seldom in a position to choose whether they will experience pathological pain. Even though pain is something that is happening within their own bodies, they do not see themselves as actively contributing to pain generation or persistence.

Clinically inflicted pain differs in one significant respect from pathological pain: it has its genesis not in the hidden and mysterious processes within the body, but in the external and visible actions of another. It may be argued that the person subjected to clinically inflicted pain has no more choice or influence on such pain than the person experiencing pathological pain. To a certain extent that is true. However, as the present study revealed, inflicted pain is different not only in terms of its origin, but also in the patient's participation in the repeated generation of such pain. By consenting to the procedures, patients gave permission to nurses (and other hospital staff) to see, touch, manipulate, and invade their bodies. Implicit in such a consent was the acceptance of the likelihood that it could result in pain and that the patient would cooperate by enduring pain in a way that would not interfere with the performance of the procedure.

The giving of consent was not a once off event for the patients. It was something they enacted through their bodies each time they underwent a painful procedure. In the patients' experience, the giving of consent required that they hand over their bodies to others to work on. This act of *handing one's body over to others* had both symbolic and lived, embodied components. For example, some patients felt invisibly changed as they walked into a treatment room or sat in the arm chair (for chemotherapy) or had the first layer of bandages removed prior to saline bath and change of dressings. They no longer felt at ease in their habitual, phenomenal bodies or free to assume postures comfortable to themselves. It was others who decided how they would sit, how their limbs would be positioned, how long they would stay still, when and how far they would move, and when the particular episode of treatment would be over.

Handing one's body over to others also entailed a bodily experience of two antithetical demands. On the one hand, patients had to allow others to do what they (others) deemed necessary, without resisting, interfering, slowing down, or preventing them from performing the treatment procedures. *Handing one's body over to others*, however, was not an act of passive giving up. It also required that the patient retain a high degree of control over his or her body in order to maintain a difficult posture, move when asked, and not cry, scream, jerk, try to withdraw, or in other ways fail to cooperate with the person performing the procedure. Trusting one's body to others and at the same time retaining a sense of personal control over the body was not easy.

In the following interview excerpt, the patient expressed the difficulties of overcoming his body's "embodied intelligence" (Benner & Wrubel, 1989, p. 42) of wanting to withdraw from pain. It required conscious effort and the restraint applied by his uninjured hand to keep his burned arm from pulling away from the nurse cleaning the wound:

> The body sort of wants to get away from it [pain] all the time. I am inclined to do anything to avoid it if possible. I guess it's being a bit of a wimp or something, but if I could avoid it I would.

Exerting control over an unwilling body, as in the above case, required conscious and determined effort. Such effort was not always successful, and the patients experienced a sense of frustration and anger toward bodies that failed them in their struggle to be cooperative. The experiences, as in the following exemplar in which the patient is describing having an arterial puncture, often led to patients feeling not only the pain of the procedure, but also a sense of estrangement from their own bodies:

> [Yesterday] I didn't want anybody around me. I just wanted to rest. But…there was this needle being pricked, and pulling, and knocking to get in. I felt sorry for her [junior doctor], but I also felt mad…angry at my own body, too.

> (Why?)

> Because I felt that I had a right to rest and [if] this body could just cooperate this time, I would be more than grateful.…Today she didn't have any trouble.…She got the blood, and I was grateful! She was grateful! So [sighs] my body behaved itself this time, for once. I hope it does so again.

Thus, it was not enough to just *hand one's body over to others*. One had to present an adequate body or accept part of the responsibility for pain that resulted from difficult and sometimes unsuccessful procedures. This was especially evident in relation to arterial and venous punctures and was therefore more commonly experienced by patients receiving intravenous chemotherapy. Patients' descriptions of unsuccessful or painful procedures were almost invariably followed by comments about their bodies or behaviors that could explain why the difficulties had occurred. In particular, patients focused on their own impaired bodies as a reason for others' difficulties or inabilities to perform a task successfully and without significant pain.

Both women with breast cancer, for example, made comments about their *impaired arms* (affected by lymphoedema) as an obstacle to nurses' work. Other patients receiving chemotherapy suggested that their veins were *too small* or had a tendency to *go into spasm* or *break down easily*. Rather than expecting nurses to recognize these difficulties as a predictable development in the course of cancer and chemotherapy, and one for which nurses should try to find solutions, patients offered apologies for presenting less than perfect bodies on which others have to work.

In a similar way, patients focused on their own behavior as another reason for unsuccessful venepunctures and experiences of pain. *Being tense* or *not relaxed enough*, failing to *drink enough* before attending the clinic, or failing to keep hands in warm water long enough for *the veins to come up* were the most frequently cited behaviors of this kind.

Nurses' questions and comments often reinforced the picture of patients' bodies as less than ideal material on which they had to work. The following exemplar is taken from field notes made during a patient's second experience of having intravenous chemotherapy:

09.50 hours:
(Nurse attempts to insert an intravenous needle. First attempt unsuccessful.)
Nurse: Missed.
Patient: That hurt! (Face becoming slightly flushed. Frowns and looks cross.)
Nurse: Your skin is really tough. I think I just pushed too hard and missed. The outside skin is too hard. Must be all that toughening up from [playing] your cricket....Do you want me to get someone else?
Patient: No! (adamant tone of voice and then concerned) You are not going to give up on me, are you?
(Receives no response)
Nurse: How much did you have to drink this morning?
Patient: Two cups of coffee.
(Again no response from the nurse who spends the next 10 minutes silently tapping patient's hand, rubbing it, coaxing a vein almost.)
Nurse: You are like a cow that will not let down its milk! (Laughs and continues tapping, rubbing, feeling for a vein.)
10.02 hours: Needle inserted successfully.

Such communication from nurses not only contributed to patients' feelings of having to accept some responsibility for the technical difficulty and painfulness of procedures performed on them, it was also a part of being constituted by the experiences of illness and treatment. People generally do not have a direct experience of their skin being *hard* or their veins being *too small* or prone to *spasms* or *breakdown*. Neither do they realize that they are apparently capable of somehow constricting their veins and making them inaccessible to a skilled nurse trying to administer their chemotherapy.

Handing one's body over to others to work on, a marred, impaired, less than perfect body, implicated patients in the generation of inflicted pain. Even if it was the actions of another that were the instruments of pain, patients' own bodies presented obstacles to a smooth and easy performance of procedures, and this, in turn, contributed to pain.

EXPECTATION AND EXPERIENCE OF BEING WOUNDED

An important aspect of inflicted pain to emerge from this study was its inextricable connection to wounding, to having one's body pierced, cut, or in some other way injured. This was an essential theme to emerge out of patients' descriptions of their experiences, but it was not evident in the nurses' accounts. Nurses tended to focus on the expected benefits of diagnostic and treatment procedures for the patients rather than on their lived experience of such procedures. Being on the receiving end of others' actions, however, gave the patients a very different appreciation of invasive and painful procedures. As in the following exemplar, in which a patient describes having a blood sample taken from his femoral artery, patients often experienced such procedures as *wounding* and the instruments used as *weapons*:

> They can fish around there, and I say "fish" literally. It should be "harpooning" because if they don't get the thing straight away they just keep jabbing and poking....There's got to be a better way to take [blood] gas samples than digging around.

> The last one took 20 minutes, and you just have to lie there as though it isn't happening to you.

Being *harpooned*, *jabbed* and *poked* and having others *digging around* one's body were painful experiences, made more difficult by the expectation that the patient would cooperate and remain still, no matter how long or painful the procedure. While the patients' lived experience was that of being wounded and suffering pain, the behavior expected from them was that of unquestioning cooperation.

In handing their bodies over to others, to treat and to wound, patients entered a particular kind of unequal relationship. To the extent that they retained any power within such a relationship, it was the power to make their bodies available to others, to cooperate with others' intentions, and to facilitate others' work. They were touched but not allowed to touch. They were handled but not allowed to handle. They were wounded but not allowed to wound in return. Nurses (and other hospital staff), on the other hand, used their own bodies to touch patients, to comfort them, to restrain them, to invade their personal space, to wound them, and even to take parts of their bodies away (as when debriding burned tissue or taking blood off for laboratory analysis).

This rather stark summation of the nature of the tactile encounter between patients and nurses might be easier to understand when it is recognized that however they felt during painful procedures patients had to remain still. To have moved, and especially to have touched a nurse performing the procedure, would have risked additional pain. Patients receiving chemotherapy, for example, were acutely aware of the risks of the intravenous needle being dislodged (and having to be reinserted) and of the drugs spilling and damaging their skin. Furthermore, nurses' gloved hands (during both chemotherapy administration and burn dressing changes) carried a clear message that they were there to perform specific technical tasks and could not at the same time be available to the patient for comfort or reassurance. While the patient's body was exposed and made available to others to work on, the nurse's body was further separated and made inaccessible by the use of gloves and in the Burn Care Unit by the use of sterile gowns and masks.

There was a particular poignancy to patients' descriptions of *being wounded* and *feeling pain* and at the same time having to control their bodily responses. Their behavior during painful procedures was marked by tension and vigilance, with the fear of wounding and harm constantly present:

When I first put the hand in Savlon™ [solution], and I actually started undressing, taking the dressing off myself, I didn't really mind that. But when it got down to the part where the hand was quite visible and very painful, then my tolerance level was quite low, and I cried…and I felt that I shouldn't be.

(Why did you feel that you shouldn't be?)

It was strange because the nurse said to me, "The injection should be working now, so you shouldn't be feeling any pain." So I felt guilty when I did feel pain…to a degree. Because the fact is that I did feel pain, and it was horrible pain.…I became very tense and very uptight, and I couldn't talk or even cry as I really wanted to.

Thus, being wounded not only caused pain, but in this context, it also required that the patient subdue her habitual bodily behaviors through which she might have expressed her pain and made the extent of her suffering known to others. The effort required to maintain such a level of self-control left patients physically tired and emotionally drained. Nevertheless, patients also experienced a sense of relief when the procedure was over and when they could once more retreat to the relative safety and comfort of their beds:

I don't know what it does, but it really makes you tired, just going through the process of washing [saline bath] and the pain going with it, and then the relief.…You know you've gone through something terrible, and you've got the relief and comfort. I don't know whether that process really takes it out of you, but it does, it really makes you tired. And you are glad to get back just to lie down and enjoy the comfort. I think it's the nonpain and knowing "Oh, this is such a relief!"

The contrast between pain and *nonpain* was an important part of the burn patients' experience. The constant possibility of wounding during painful procedures and the ensuing feelings of vulnerability meant that they could not relax and passively allow others to work on them. They were active participants in the procedure, tense, vigilant, and as far as possible cooperative.

The connection between *wounding* and *pain* was reinforced in several ways. During chemotherapy, for example, patients were warned about the damage the drugs would cause to local tissues if the needle was not positioned properly or the solution leaked out. They were asked to tell the nurse if they experienced any discomfort or pain, particularly any sensations of *burning*, *stinging*, or *heat* along the vein being injected. Such requests for feedback were experienced as reassuring, a sign that nurses would pay heed to patient's self-reports and not continue an obviously painful procedure. At the same time, they contributed to patients' *expectations of wounding and pain* and made it more difficult to use distraction as a way of coping with the situation. The need to maintain vigilance added to the feelings of both tension and vulnerability.

Patients with burn injuries often talked about feeling *vulnerable* and *exposed* during treatment procedures. In contrast to the safety of their beds, undergoing dressing changes opened the patients to two dangers: the danger of being wounded and marred beyond the initial injuries and the danger of pain resulting from this new wounding. As in the following exemplar, where the patient is describing removal of dressings and a saline bath in preparation for her first skin grafting operation, the temporary safety of the person's bed could never be taken for granted:

It was painful and cold. I really wanted to be back in the security of my bed. I didn't really want to be out in the open. I felt very, very unfeminine. Not just because my body was exposed...it's hard to explain....It was very cold, and it seemed to take an awfully long time, much longer than I thought it would....I was worrying about what was going to happen and what was really left of me....Scary. Very vulnerable.

Particular techniques and modes of treatment often added to patients' fears of *wounding and pain* and the perceptions of medical instruments as *weapons*. This was particularly evident in the Oncology Clinic, with the use of peripheral veins and administration of chemotherapy by slow intravenous injection using a series of large syringes. It was not at all unusual for a nurse to place a tray with six or more syringes, several of the 20 cc size, on a table next to the patient before proceeding to insert the intravenous needle. In the words of one patient,

It was frightening, it really was. To see that many syringes and how big they were as well. It is off-putting.

Such "horse syringes" were seen by patients as disproportionately large in relation to the small veins in their hands through which all the fluid would have to be injected, which added to their feelings of vulnerability and their *fears of wounding*. Such fears were not speculative but grounded in patients' own embodied experiences of procedures and how much they had hurt in the past. The speed at which the solution was injected was particularly important:

One of the nurses did say one day, "You've got lovely big veins!" and was busy pumping the stuff in. Well, that to my mind was the most uncomfortable session I've had with them because I think she was inclined to be a little bit eager with it, just pushing it in a little bit fast.

In fact, there was considerable variation between staff in terms of the time taken to administer chemotherapy. On the whole, nurses tended to take considerably longer than physicians to inject similar volumes of fluid. In the case of one patient, for example, on a particular occasion a nurse took 25 minutes to administer 112 mls of solution. On two subsequent visits, a medical registrar took 9 and 7 minutes, respectively, to administer the same drugs in the same volume of fluid to the same patient. The result was not only stinging pain at the conclusion of the latter two procedures, but also, following the last procedure, an extensive area of local inflammation, which produced ongoing pain, took over 3 months to heal, and required medical intervention. This damage to local tissues also limited the number of peripheral veins available for subsequent intravenous injections, in turn contributing to a greater number of unsuccessful venepunctures as this patient's chemotherapy continued.

Being wounded and having pain inflicted was something that patients experienced directly in their bodies. They also thought about the experience, reflected on it, and interpreted it within their particular situation, thus giving it meaning and making it more tolerable (or in some instances, more distressing). What should not be overlooked or minimized, however, is the impact of the direct experience through which each person gained embodied knowledge of the unpleasant, hurting quality of such *wounding and pain* and a fresh awareness of the inborn desire for safety and comfort. Hence, during each new procedure, patients experienced physical tension and vigilance in anticipation of pain and wounding. At the same time, they had to exert conscious control over their bodies, handing them over to others as objects on which others could work unimpeded.

The patients' lived experience of *being wounded and having pain* was a potent reminder of their existence as embodied beings. Yet, at the same time, it contained within it a demand to deny the taken-for-granted, lived familiarity with the body and its embodied intelligence, which would have protected them from further harm. Instead, in the midst of pain, these people had to consciously and deliberately try not to react with their habitual bodies: They had to avoid withdrawing, pushing away, hitting back, and preventing others from wounding them further. In essence, consenting to painful procedures, to *being wounded and having pain inflicted*, was not so much an act of will as it was a series of bodily events of self-denial and self-control achieved *by* the body as much as *through* the body. In the process, patients in pain found themselves restrained in their bodily actions and, even more specifically, in their vocal expressions of their experience.

RESTRAINING THE BODY AND THE VOICE

One of the essential features of inflicted pain is that it takes place in a social context; it is experienced in the presence of others. The conflicting demands of being wounded (and wanting to withdraw from the source of such wounding) and of having to hand one's body over to others to work on limit the possibilities of how patients live through and endure clinically inflicted pain.

Living through and enduring inflicted pain for the patients in this study meant learning to let go of at least some of their habitual responses and finding new ways of being in the situation. Not being able to withdraw from others, specifically those inflicting the pain, was the crucial restriction, which in turn limited the range of expressions or behaviors the person in pain could use to endure inflicted pain. Thus, while pulling back from the source of pain, hitting back in retaliation, swearing, cursing, yelling or screaming were recognized by patients as habitual ways of responding to pain, particularly pain inflicted in work or sports accidents or in physical fights with others, they also recognized that these behaviors were not the behaviors that they could or should use in response to clinically inflicted pain. Instead, patients felt a very strong need to *retain composure* and to *be cooperative*. Even crying or moaning as a means of letting-go and releasing tension and expressing pain were no longer accepted as appropriate. The patients felt they were constrained and not free to express their experiences. They were acutely aware that their habitual, spontaneous, taken-for-granted being in the world had to be replaced by a constant effort to restrain their bodily actions and their vocal expressions. The categories of "body and voice" (Scarry, 1985, p. 182) most accurately capture the focus of patients' efforts in maintaining composure and being cooperative.

In the following exemplar, a patient, unable to control his habitual inclination to use expletives loudly when in severe pain, describes the importance and the difficulty of retaining composure. Faced with a need to express his pain while at the same time retaining control and behaving in a socially acceptable manner, this patient invented a new vocabulary:

> The stitches [being removed from a new skin graft] were just a very, very sharp pain. If it hadn't stopped...I probably would have yelled out, or something. It was sharp. It was enough to make you want to cry out, which reminds me, I've invented a lot of new words.

(Like what?)

Oh, a lot of new words. It's a new language really. It's not swearing, it's nothing. You can't swear [in this situation]. So I've got a few new words that only I know the meaning of. Just a way of expressing pain rather than yelling out.

The presence of others required that habitual ways of coping be restrained. For this patient, to have cried or used expletives would have indicated that he was in pain and that he was experiencing difficulties in tolerating what was being done to him. But additionally, and perhaps more important, it would have called into question the nurses' right to inflict pain in the course of their work, and it would have called into question their skills and abilities when causing as much pain as they did. However difficult and exhausting the enduring, it was what patients felt they had to go through and *put up with*.

By their patient and, as far as possible, silent endurance, patients accepted inflicted pain as legitimate and justified, as something beyond their control. Others could both cause pain and decide what analgesic medication would be given, if any, but the patients' duty was to endure. Pain was the price of being healed, and it had to be paid:

I am injured, and I want to get well. I want to be cured and if that nurse wants to do this or that to cure me…no matter what it is, she's got to be able to do it. She's got to be allowed to do that. It's no good saying, "Now, you are not doing that! It hurts too much, you can't do it."…If it's going to hurt, if you can get a little injection that will prevent the pain, cracker! But…if for some reason or other I couldn't have any [pain relief] I would be prepared to grit my teeth and hope I could put up with it.

Thus, living through and enduring inflicted pain meant *having to restrain one's voice* as well as *having to restrain one's habitual body*. The full extent of one's pain and suffering could not be expressed to others, particularly not to those inflicting the pain. This restraint was especially evident in the efforts patients with burns expended trying not to cry, scream, or in other ways give voice to their pain during prolonged painful procedures. To have done so would not have been socially acceptable since neither nurses nor patients accepted free vocal expression as appropriate, even when in severe pain. For the patients in pain, it would also have signalled loss of all control in the situation, including control over their communication with their world. When already naked and having their wounded and marred bodies exposed, to be then reduced to preverbal cries and screams was also to lose their fragile sense of dignity and worth as human beings.

It is only by recognizing the enormity of the losses facing patients during painful procedures that the effort they made to stay in control, no matter how painful the experience, becomes clearer. To retain a sense of control, they used a variety of approaches, among them prayer, objectifying pain and giving it shape and personality, as well as, very physical behaviors such as gritting their teeth or holding tight on to the bed or someone's hand if that was available. Often, as in the following exemplars, these approaches were combined:

> I prayed a lot, and I think that is a major thing that got me up and about....And also myself, the physical person that I am, that also helped a bit....When you get pain and you feel hurt...that gives me a buzz and makes me fight it....I am the energetic sort of guy as you know, and that is part and parcel of me that gets me going to fight this thing. Plus a bit of prayer and getting help from the Lord....That guy [pain] is history because he is going down.

> I suppose the Panadol™ that I asked for at a particular time [helped]. And sort of gritting my teeth, just really biting hard on my teeth. That helped....Especially when they put that white cream on my arm just the other day. I just gritted my teeth, and then in time the pain went. And a little prayer of course. I usually say a little quiet prayer to myself.

Unlike nurses, patients seldom used the term *coping* when describing their living through experiences of pain. Rather, they talked of *putting up with* and *enduring* pain and of *going through* or *handling* frightening or painful events. They considered that they had done so successfully when, in the midst of pain, they were able to retain a sense of composure, in other words, when they were *able to restrain their bodies and their voices*.

The impact of pain-relieving medication was also experienced as reassurance because the medication would make it easier to control the body and the voice. In the following exemplar, the patient is commenting on the effects of receiving an intravenous injection of Morphine prior to a large dressing change:

> I liked that because to me there is less pain. It's going to cut the level so that I've got only the level of 2 [on a 10-point scale], instead of 7 or 8....To know that you can sit there and they can tear all those bandages off. I shouldn't really use the word "tear"...take all your bandages

off, and you are not going to feel it. That's great, marvellous! It does a lot for your own confidence, I suppose. You can lie or sit there, as the case may be. This quiet confidence that you are not going to get hurt, you are not going to be yelling and screaming.

Just as they experienced feelings of vulnerability and threats of wounding, patients also experienced challenges to their confidence, that is, that they would be able to retain their composure and exert adequate control over their bodies and voices. For the patients receiving chemotherapy, this occurred with increasing frequency as chemotherapy progressed and the incidence of unsuccessful venepunctures and complications related to chemotherapy increased. Patients spoke about having to endure several attempts at needle insertion as *reducing them to tears*. This was a particularly apt description of situations in which they not only lacked words to express their distress, but also lost their composure.

Composure was a way in which patients presented themselves as being in control of their bodies and their voices in a difficult situation. It was different from the unself-conscious way of being in a familiar situation. Maintaining composure required a great deal of effort, preparatory rehearsal as to what would happen and how the person would handle impending events, and expectation that others would not significantly change the situation for which the person had prepared. When one of these factors was lacking, such as when a patient was too tired and unable to sustain the necessary effort, the body and the voice could not be restrained and composure would be lost. In the following exemplar, the patient was explaining why she felt unable to agree to a surgical procedure on the day it was suggested:

You know exactly what you are going to experience when you get there, and you steel yourself, at the same time putting on a very brave face. Only one thing needs to go wrong and straight away, it's very hard to handle it all. My first instance was when they wanted me to have that debridement [of the ulcerating breast tumor, with initial suggestion that it should be done under a local anaesthetic]. He said, "Straight away," and of course I said, "Today!? Today!?" I was in a panic because I didn't know I was going to have that and that was a whole new ball game to me.

I felt I'd had enough that day...I didn't expect that happening....It was a bit of a shock to think that suddenly I had to go through something else....I didn't think I could have coped with it that day because I'd had enough with the chemo [earlier that morning]....You always think that you may feel it if you are awake, and I thought to myself, "If it is done under local, then obviously they will put some injections up somewhere around the breast," and I thought that could be quite painful.

They were things I hadn't planned on having to handle, and therefore I found that that did upset me quite a bit....You retain a bit of composure, but it is much harder to retain it and inside you end up in a bit of turmoil.

Retaining composure was part of *restraining the body and the voice.* Composure made it possible for patients to present their bodies for others to work on, despite expectations and experiences of wounding and pain. It allowed nurses and others to go on performing painful procedures, often without being aware how much pain they were inflicting in a particular situation. It also allowed patients to retain a sense of personal intactness in situations in which they felt marred and different.

The essential nature of clinically inflicted pain is that it not only results from actions of another, but that much of it must be endured in the presence of another. Yet what the experience of the patients in this study has shown is that the greatest impact of having to suffer pain in the presence of those who have inflicted it was to restrain the expression of such pain. The nurses' presence sometimes served as a witness to patients' pain and as a means to prevent, minimize, and relieve the intensity and impact of such pain. But much more commonly nurses' presence served to restrain patients' expressions of their pain and limited their range of choices of being in the situation.

By *restraining the body and the voice,* patients retain a sense of dignity as well as a certain sense of control and intactness in the situation. At the same time, they lose the power inherent in human voice of making others take notice and thus of altering the situation. When present, the voice demands that it be heard and that its meaning be taken into account in defining a situation. The absence of voice, on the other hand, permits those inflicting pain to define the encounter in terms that frequently disregard the lived experience of the person in pain. Thus, *restraining the body and the voice* facilitates the technical performance of painful procedures, but at the same time, it makes the patient's experience of pain and distress in the situation even more private and unshareable.

In the process of living through repeated episodes of inflicted pain, patients face the tasks of not only enduring the immediate situation, but also of coming to terms with their own experience as well as with the actions of those who inflict pain. In phenomenological terms, patients are 'oriented' toward their lifeworld and 'intentionally' involved in it (Merleau-Ponty, 1962; van Manen, 1990). This involvement in their lifeworld, the constituting and the being constituted by the experience of inflicted pain, is the subject of the next chapter.

Chapter 5
The Lifeworld Of Inflicted Pain: Patients' Perceptions Of Others, Pain, And Self

Living through experiences of clinically inflicted pain requires patients to deal with the imperatives of such pain: the need to *hand one's body over to others, the wounding, the restraining of the body and the voice,* and, always, *the inherent painfulness and hurt of pain.* These essential themes of the embodied nature of inflicted pain were presented in the last chapter. My aim in this chapter is to expand the picture and to consider the "lifeworld" (van Manen, 1990, p. 182) of inflicted pain, the world of the immediate experience that involves the patient and the nurse, the tactile encounter through which pain is generated, and the impact of the pain on the patient. Phenomenological concern with embodiment continues in this chapter and is expanded to consider "the situation" (Benner & Wrubel, 1989, p. 80), the socially meaningful environment within which patients encounter those who inflict pain and within which they come to terms with their experiences.

Patient-participants in this study spoke about the difficulties and demands of living with the immediacy and the severity of inflicted pain. But they had other concerns also. They were aware of their need for treatment and of the basic human need for care and comfort. They were also aware of the impact that others' actions had on their embodied being, and they were aware of their own altered sense of place and time. Thus, to understand inflicted pain as a lived human experience, it is necessary to go beyond the essential themes discussed so far while at the same time returning to them and to the context of the experience.

PATIENTS' PERCEPTIONS OF THOSE WHO INFLICT PAIN

People who experience inflicted pain also experience the presence of those whose actions generate such pain. They have to live through pain and, at the same time, live through a series of encounters with others during which their bodies are exposed and handed over to others. What the patients in this study came to appreciate was that the public domain of their pain experience left them both exposed to others and yet alone. In the main, their public exposure was not to fellow sufferers but to those who inflicted the pain, those who could not in any direct way share the experience of being in pain and having to endure it. Thus, despite the presence of others, patients felt alone in their experience, or as one patient expressed it,

No matter how kind people are, you go through it on your own. There is only yourself that can go through it and handle it.

The feelings of being alone occurred not because the experience of pain was private, but because the nature of others' presence was such that it exposed patients to possibilities of wounding and pain that only patients could feel. Rather than offering a sense of privacy and thus safety from others' actions, the feelings of being alone had the effect of isolating the person in the midst of a social situation. This sense of being alone occurred despite the fact that it was the tactile and often physically invasive nature of the encounter with others that resulted in pain being inflicted and having to be endured. What stood out in the patients' descriptions of the nurses who cared for them and administered their treatments was the quality of their touch. The interactions that left the deepest impression on patients were those that involved them in a tactile encounter with nurses. It was through the quality of nurses' touch that patients sensed how a particular procedure might go, how vigilant they would need to remain, and how much effort they would have to expend on living through the experience.

The quality of the tactile encounter

Touching another human being can occur for a variety of reasons and with a variety of intentions. In the nurse-patient interaction, it is often used to comfort, reassure, and communicate care. For the patients receiving intravenous chemotherapy or undergoing treatment following burn injuries, however, nurses' touch had a much more instrumental purpose. In their experience, nurses' touch was associated with treatment procedures and only very seldom was it perceived as an expression of empathy, comforting, or reassurance. Most often, it was a means of accomplishing treatment procedures and was often mediated by instruments and other material objects. Thus, what patients experienced was not only the actions of nurses' bodies on their own bodies, but actions of nurses' bodies mediated by needles, forceps, spatula, jets of water directed from a nozzle, and the stripping and application of wound dressings.

As discussed earlier, patients often experienced painful procedures as wounding and medical instruments as weapons. Yet they seldom talked about the instrument itself; rather, their references were to the person using the instrument and the quality of the person's actions. Their lack of control over others' actions made the patients especially aware of the differences in how others touched, handled, and acted on their bodies. Thus, patients were acutely aware that individual nurses varied not only in their attitudes to pain relief and pain management, but that they also varied in their basic approach to the patient and their handling of the patient's body. This was especially so for the patients with burn injuries.

The very touch of each nurse had a quality that could engender feelings of comfort and trust or, on the other hand, a sense of unease, tension and vigilance. Nurses varied in the amount of pain they inflicted and in the way they influenced individual patient's perceived capacity to endure the pain. What stood out in patients' descriptions of nurses and their assessment of nursing work was the quality of the tactile encounter:

> I've noticed a big difference in the nurses, the way in which they take a situation. Every nurse has a different touch, a different feel....There are two nurses that I could say do have a very gentle and a very soothing, relaxing feel, but there are also two who I would cringe [to see] at the door because I know what their feel is like. The first one I had on Saturday [had] a very gentle feeling....I didn't have my eyes open either, but it was very relaxing and a very soothing, cool sort of feeling. But also the touch was very, very gentle and it was very relaxing. She was talking to me at the same time, too. And she was very careful....It just helped me to relax. In my own way, I think it stopped my body from tensing.

The intimate nature of tactile encounters meant that nurses' actions had a direct and significant impact on the embodied experience of the patient.

As in the above exemplar, a particular touch had a particular feel. The experience of being touched (the feeling of being touched) in turn spread through the body, producing either feelings of safety and relaxation or feelings of tension and vigilance. Even though patients tolerated, with varying amounts of effort, whatever was inflicted on them, their lived experience was altered significantly by the actions of different nurses. Two contrasting categories of nurses emerged from patients' descriptions of their experiences: *the good nurses*, who patients hoped would be the ones assigned to care for them, especially on the days when painful procedures were scheduled; and *the good-but nurses*, who were more likely to engender feelings of concern and expectations of wounding and pain. Thus, nurses were evaluated principally in terms of their capacity to ameliorate or exacerbate pain, and pain became the core variable around which these judgements were made.

The good nurses

There was a high degree of consensus among patients as to the qualities of nurses whom they identified as *good nurses*. Such nurses could be trusted to not only perform the necessary procedures with skill and technical expertise, but to act with sensitivity and awareness of the impact their actions would have on the particular patient. The essential qualities that led patients in the Burn Care Unit to regard a nurse as a good nurse were:

- *Gentleness*: A quality of touch and physical handling of the patient's body characterized by *softness, tenderness,* attentiveness to specific, particularly sensitive or painful parts of the patient's body, and an overriding concern for patient's comfort;

- *Trustworthiness*: A complex set of characteristics that included *calmness* as well as a capacity to *inspire confidence* and reduce vigilance by making it possible for a patient to relax even in the midst of a painful procedure. Nurses who kept their promises to stop when the pain became severe and to provide additional pain relief were regarded as trustworthy;

- *Sensitivity*: A quality of *attending* to particular patients, focusing on their experience and their feelings in the situation, including knowing when to talk and when to use silence, and *pacing* a procedure according to the patient's capacity to tolerate it;

- *Technical competence*: A quality of being *organized, efficient,* and able to perform technical tasks with skill and agility. It also included the ability to be *systematic* and *methodical* in the performance of technically intricate tasks; and

- *Knowledge and skillful communication:* A quality of not only knowing what information a particular patient would find helpful at a particular time, but also having the ability to communicate it in such a way that the patient felt informed, reassured and encouraged.

A nurse with these qualities had not only knowledge and skills, but knew how and when to use them, making each patient feel special, cared for, encouraged and reassured. The nurse's success in achieving a particular quality of being-with the patient, and especially a particular quality of tactile encounter, became a part of the patient's embodied experience of treatment and of pain. The following exemplars capture vividly the impact that *good nurses* had on the patients and on their experience of difficult and often painful procedures:

I think I said the other day that there's good nurses....[They] know how to put a bandage on, know how to give an injection, this sort of thing...and I've been thinking about that a wee bit, and I think a lot of it is attitude. It's the way they approach the task that they are actually doing, whether it's wrapping a hand or stripping a bandage. Naturally, most of the more senior nurses should be better because they are more experienced, but it's not always the case...just the way they approach you, the attitude toward it. A good nurse seems to go to the job and do it and know exactly what she is doing...have a system, a method...she has done it before. And if she is cleaning off a hand, she will start from the small fingers and work away through to the thumb....The little things like...when they are pulling the skin off. Some of them just get it and they just pull it—the way they want. Or in other cases, a couple of nurses, they give it small pulls, see which way it is going to go, then they'll pull the way the skin wants to go. They don't pull the way that they want to go, which is half the pain. If the skin is allowed to go the way it wants, it's got to come off anyway so why not let it go the way it wants to go? And it's a lot less painful.

She was lovely because she was very tender...she got all the dead skin off and really wiped it and talked to me the whole time. We talked about other things, but at the same time she was doing it and I was watching everything, the progress that was going on, and she was explaining things to me. That's what I liked about her. She really explained things to me and what was happening. Because to me it was just like a big mess, and she said, "Oh no, look, your skin is taking and there are just these parts that haven't healed."...So she was telling me all those kinds of things and was really lovely.

Technical competence exercised in the context of a caring interaction, with as much attention to the person as to the procedure being performed, was recognized and deeply appreciated by the patients. What made a difference to the patients' experience was the nurses' ability to integrate their quality of *being-with* the patient with the quality of their *acting-on* the patient. Such an approach did not render the procedure painless, but it did make it easier for patients to hand their bodies over, and it reduced the threat of wounding and the fear that the pain would become intolerable. Far too frequently, however, what patients experienced was an altogether different approach, leading to a very different experience.

The good-but nurses

Just as there was a high degree of consensus as to the qualities of *the good nurses*, there was considerable agreement about specific actions that patients found intensely, and perhaps unnecessarily, painful. However, despite such distressingly painful experiences, which they did attribute to nurses' actions, patients were reluctant to name the nurse or nurses involved. Their comments about particularly painful procedures were usually qualified with statements about nurses' positive attributes. Often the positive comments came first and then were followed by descriptions of events that presented the nurse in quite a different light. Thus, the term *the good-but nurses* is used here to refer to the nurses whom patients perceived as capable and at other times caring, but at the same time, they felt that these nurses lacked the qualities of the truly *good nurses*. As shown in the following exemplar, patients who were in pain and knew that the procedures they were about to undergo would be painful felt particularly vulnerable when assigned to *good-but nurses*:

I struck one who I thought was really rough....She is an excellent nurse because I had her again later. But...I think when you are really in pain you need someone with a very gentle touch, and she was very firm. She was very firm, and she plastered the [silver sulphadiazine™] cream on, you know. It was painful, and it was the first time I had really experienced pain when the cream was put on. I was going out that day, and she left all my fingers exposed....There was no cream put on those...and they were in pain; they were sore. That's why I thought she is all right when you are a bit better. But not really when you are going through that pain. She is a very good bandager and she is very clean, and she cares but not when a patient is in pain. I didn't think that she would be suitable for that.

For the patient who is very painful, it is most important I think to get a nurse who is very tender and very soft. That's how I felt anyhow.

Like the procedures they performed, *the good-but nurses* could not be avoided. Patients did not feel able to challenge nurses who had hurt them in the past, for example, by requesting that another nurse attend to them or by asking that the nurse act differently, except to perhaps warn them of particularly tender spots and hope that they would be more careful as the result. The essential characteristics of these *good-but nurses* were as follows:

- *Roughness*: The quality of touch or physical contact with the patient, including *firm, scraping, hard* motions while in contact with burn wounds. Roughness involved not only a quality of touch, but also insensitivity to its impact and disregard for the person treated in such a way;

- *Unpredictability*: A quality of being inconsistent and lacking dependability and trustworthiness so that patients, unsure of how they might be treated, experienced tension, worry and vigilance, feeling uncertain or fearful about the impact of the nurses' actions on them;

- *Disregard for the individual patient*: A quality of attentiveness to the technical task to the exclusion of sensitivity to the particular patient. It included persisting with the task and the particular approach to it, regardless of how the patient might be responding. One patient summed up a nurse who lacked this sensitivity to the individual patient as *very thorough, but not quite with me*;

- *Limited technical competence*: A quality of being able to accomplish the necessary tasks but in a mechanical way, without awareness of how to work with the structures of the body or of the impact of the actions on the embodied person. One patient described this lack of technical perceptiveness as being *like* [a carpenter] *going against the grain in timber. If you plane it, it's a lot harder going against the grain than it is with it*; and

- *Restricted communication*: A quality of being unwilling or unable to respond to patients' needs for information, reassurance, or encouragement. Nurses showed this by becoming uncommunicative while focused on the technical tasks or by introducing irrelevant conversation topics.

While nurses who exhibited such qualities were in a minority, their impact on patients was far greater than their numbers. A physically rough and apparently uncaring approach at a time when patients felt particularly vulnerable and easily hurt could produce fears and concerns that were difficult to overcome. Patients were especially aware of the feelings of vulnerability and tension that these experiences created and the energy that they needed in order to live through them. The last exemplar captured one patient's experience of pain resulting from actions that the patient knew did not need to hurt as much as they did. This knowledge was not enough to prevent such an experience from being repeated, hence the feelings of vulnerability and the need for vigilance.

The speed with which a procedure was performed could also impact on the amount of pain experienced by the patient, as shown in the next exemplar. Again, however, one can sense that it is the nurse's attitude to the patient that is as much at issue as the speed with which the nurse had acted. The patient is left feeling not only pain, but also a sense of having been disregarded, of feeling that he did not matter as a person:

> Some nurses take their time about what they do so that they don't inflict too much pain, and some nurses just rush it. They just want the dressing over and done with and go on to work with someone else....I can remember one nurse, she cut the dressing off and just ripped it clean off my back, and that had me in pain for about half an hour. Even though I was in a saline bath, trying to relax, I could still feel the pain. That was the first time I had taken the saline bath without having a Morphine shot, and so the pain stuck with me for quite a while.

The second exemplar is provided by a patient who contrasted her earlier experience of being treated by a particularly sensitive nurse who alleviated her fears, helped her to relax and made her feel special and cared for with the experience of a nurse who seemed to be almost the complete opposite. The result was more pain, more tension, and more energy expended on dealing with the procedure and its aftermath:

> It hurt. It definitely hurt. It's hard to describe how it hurt, but it did not have the same calming, soothing effect because I almost felt that she was in a hurry. She was coming from one patient to another, and

to another, and I was one [of] perhaps five or six....The feel was very rushed and not relaxed. I felt quite tense when she left here, and it took me actually quite a while to relax and to get back into a relaxed state. Quite a while. I noticed that particularly today...it's had an effect on how badly I've tolerated pain. I haven't tolerated pain particularly well today....It just made me more uptight, made me more tense and therefore made it more difficult to cope.

What also made coping more difficult for patients in the Burn Care Unit was the unpredictability concerning which of the 30 nurses working there would be assigned to them on a particular day. They could not ask for a particular nurse and often had to cope with new nurses, that is, nurses who had not treated their wounds or had not done so recently. Without an ongoing knowledge of patients' wounds, "new" nurses lacked an adequate awareness of the areas that were healing, had become infected, or were particularly sensitive and therefore had to be touched with extreme care. This lack of continuity limited nurses' ability to develop trust with patients, thus increasing patients' feelings of vulnerability and the need for vigilance.

The much smaller number of nurses in the Oncology Clinic meant that over time patients became familiar with the nurses and had their chemotherapy administered by a person who knew them. Overall, the Oncology Clinic nurses were regarded as *nice, friendly,* and *competent.* As discussed earlier, patients with cancer often accepted responsibility for unsuccessful venepunctures and resulting pain, seeing the cause not in the actions of others but in their own damaged bodies. Nevertheless, they, too, came across those, most often laboratory staff, who hurt them more than their past experience had taught them was necessary. In the following exemplar, the patient is recalling being faced by an unfamiliar laboratory technician on a routine visit to the laboratory and the ensuing experience of a particularly painful venepuncture:

She saw me in the corridor and said, "Oh, there is nobody else here. I'll do you." And she proceeded to *do* me. And *that hurt*. She did hurt. It is only putting the needle in, but she hurt. She didn't seem to get the needle right....I didn't really study what she was doing....I am not overenthusiastic about watching people doing that to me...but I did watch her because she hurt. I don't think she spent enough time trying to raise the vein to the point where she could get the needle in easily....I thought she had gone past the vein. And I think what she was doing was searching for it under the skin with the needle in, rather than have another go for it. I've always felt...if they couldn't make it the first time [it would be better] if they took the needle out and tried somewhere else. I've always felt that the ones that caused the problems were the ones that...searched for the vein under the skin after they've got the needle in.

As with the patients with burns, the patients with cancer came to know those who worked on them largely through the quality of the tactile encounter. Trusting their bodies to others, handing themselves over to be wounded and hurt, as well as, living with uncertainty about how a procedure may go and how much pain they would have to endure were essential parts of their lived experience. Despite the wounding and the pain, and despite experiences with nurses and other staff who added to their pain and suffering, patients continued with their treatments. To do so they had to find meaning and purpose in what was happening to them.

CONSTITUTING THE EXPERIENCE OF INFLICTED PAIN AND GIVING IT MEANING

Throughout life, people constitute their experiences by becoming involved in them, interpreting them and giving them meaning, and in turn, they are constituted by them by being changed in their understanding and experience of themselves and of their world (Benner & Wrubel, 1989). Experiences of injury, illness and pain seem to demand that those involved in them reflect not only on sensations inherent in these experiences, but also on their meanings in the context of the person's life and situation. While the focus here is on inflicted pain, it is not possible to entirely separate the experience of pain from the context of injury and illness in which pain is experienced. For the patients in this study, the experience of injury and illness stimulated a search for meaning, while pain added a certain sense of urgency to the quest.

In the early stages, patients conceived their situation in punitive terms, with both illness and pain as *punishment* for something they could not quite grasp. For some, the sense of being punished was strong; for others, there was a less focused sense of unease and search for explanation. In either case, the questions mostly started with a "why": "Why cancer" or "burn injuries?" "Why me?" "Why does it have to hurt so much?" "Why does the pain not go away?" Such questions were not satisfied by technical explanations. Instead, they reflected a concern with the metaphysical, a concern with the nature of the taken-for-granted world in which pain and suffering might not have been given much consideration previously and that had to be questioned and understood from a fresh vantage point. Later, patients accepted pain as an *unavoidable part of treatment*, which highlighted their lack of control in the situation and their dependence on others. In the end, patients were able to endure repeated episodes of inflicted pain by seeing them as unavoidable while at the same time continuing to ask questions, including questions to which there were no ready answers. Thus, there was no single meaning attached to the experience of inflicted pain. Rather, meanings were embedded in the broader context of patients' experience and changed as their treatment progressed and other circumstances altered.

Pain as *punishment*

Whether they regarded it as *fair* or *unfair, deserved* or *undeserved, meaningful* or *making no sense at all*, patients often talked about the early phases of illness and initial encounters with pain as *punishment* or as a *trial* to be endured. It was part of the bewilderment in the face of personal tragedy, part of seeking for meaning in a situation that seemed devoid of meaning, and part of trying to identify the source of control over the lives that were no longer under their personal control. To be punished means to have to submit to someone else's power, to be subjected to pain and deprivation of another's making, and to be restricted in the exercise of personal will. Some patients were certain of their innocence and the injustice of the punishment inflicted on them. One patient, for example, had strong feelings of anger at the injustice of what was happening to her as well as a strong sense of the interrelatedness of injuries, pain, and her response to the situation in which she found herself. Her *punishment* was a rude shock, a violence done to her and her body that she did not expect or feel that she deserved:

I don't think it was fair what happened. I don't think I deserved that....I've never ever thought that this would happen, never, never, never ever! Never!...It is usually the physical pain that sets my emotions going and...usually they'll make me look at what's happened, and when I look at what's happened, I think about what's happened, and then, when I think about what's happened, I cry. So it's all interrelated.

This is another body that I don't know. Not me. I don't deserve it. It's not me. I don't deserve it. I've been saying that to myself all day. And I was hoping that it will go away.

Other patients seemed to accept the notion of some cosmic system of justice in which punishment follows improper actions, regardless of whether the person is or is not aware of personal wrongdoing:

I thought I must have done something wrong as to why I was being punished with a cancer....Perhaps I...I don't know, just smoked too much or something, or drunk too much or something. But I don't drink, and I don't smoke that much. I've got to stop, stop or cut down, or stop. I don't drink, but I just wonder what the hell I've done.

Patients could rage at the injustice of undeserved *punishment*, search for likely causes in their past or present behaviors, or question the reasons for the situation in which they found themselves. What they did not question was the right of nurses and others to perform invasive and painful procedures, no matter how intense the pain. Patients with cancer and those with burn injuries both saw their situation as one in which they had no other choice than to endure what others decided was necessary. No matter how intense and difficult to tolerate, pain that resulted from *necessary* procedures was accepted as something that they as individuals could not avoid.

Necessary procedures and *unavoidable* pain

If one were to take a philosophical perspective, it could be argued that the procedures performed on the patients who participated in this study were not of themselves either *necessary* or *unavoidable*. They were not sought for their own sake. Rather, in seeking to be healed, patients were faced with these procedures as the means toward the goal of *becoming themselves again*. If the medical attention had not been sought, then the necessity and unavoidability of the painful procedures would not have arisen, although other consequences would have followed and become unavoidable. Even from the clinical practice perspective, however, the procedures are not always necessary or unavoidable. For example, the number and frequency of venepunctures performed on patients with cancer could have been reduced by the use of a central vein catheter or by the use of one vein and a single puncture to withdraw blood for laboratory analysis and to administer the chemotherapy. There are technical reasons as to why one option may be considered as more appropriate than another, but the point is that there are options. Similarly, there are options related to the type of dressings applied to burn wounds and the consequent frequency of dressing changes and the pain involved in their performance.

What stands out from the patients' descriptions of their experience in this study is their perception of a complete lack of options and choices and their acceptance of others as experts whose decisions could not be challenged. No matter how traumatic, wounding, and painful to endure, procedures through which diagnostic information was obtained and treatments carried out were accepted by patients as *necessary*. Even though they realized that such procedures could be carried out with varying degrees of pain, patients expected *some* pain and could not predict with any certainty how much pain they would experience on any given occasion. Some degree of pain was, therefore, seen as *unavoidable*. Yet, however necessary the procedure and however justified the pain, inflicted pain was something that patients considered as intrinsically bad, destructive, and something they wished could be avoided. In the following interview extract, a patient who endured her pain with considerable stoicism and outward composure nevertheless summed up her experience as

> traumatic! I hope it never happens to me again. I know now how it feels when people get burnt. You don't realize the pain that they go through until you have been through it....I only wish they could do it [get burns to heal] without pain.

It was the realization that *they* (nurses) had to act on the patient's body to effect recovery that shaped patients' perceptions of painful procedures as necessary. Yet however necessary the procedure, the associated pain was something they would rather have avoided and wished to avoid in the future. Thus, while patients endured inflicted pain as something they personally could not avoid, they did not accept it as either intrinsically good or an absolute benefit to them. Even as they recognized the inextricable connection between certain procedures and inflicted pain, patients made a distinction between the procedures that they hoped would rid their bodies of cancer or help their burned bodies to heal and the pain that came with the procedures. Such pain was not so much accepted as endured, and then not because it was seen as necessary or beneficial, but because *it could not be avoided*. This perception contrasted sharply with the perceptions of nurses, many of whom regarded *inflicted pain* as not only *necessary*, but also as *beneficial*.

Patients' perceptions of procedures as *necessary* and of inflicted pain as *unavoidable* were reinforced by nurses and other staff who offered no alternative explanations. The prevailing message was that what was being done was what needed to be done and the way it was being done was either the only way or the best way it could be done. Thus, if patients felt pain, it was because pain could not be avoided. In this context, patients with burn injuries had little perception or understanding of undertreatment for pain, that is, of not being given appropriate analgesic medication in sufficient dosage and frequency to produce a significant reduction in pain. What the patients reported was varying levels of pain and not infrequently intense and prolonged pain. Despite such pain, however, they did not challenge nurses or doctors in relation to the analgesic medication provided or the way in which procedures were performed. Also, patients did not mention whether nurses were able to adequately manage the pain using analgesic drugs or other measures. Rather, their descriptions were of pain that had to be endured. As illustrated by one patient, an intramuscular injection of Morphine could prevent severe pain, but if it was not given, then the nurses' judgement would go unchallenged and the patient would "grit his teeth and hope he could put up with the pain." Because the procedure was *necessary*, the pain was *unavoidable* and therefore endured, with only rare requests for pain relief and no sense that the experience could have been different:

> What made it painful for me was the peeling of the blisters and the water concentrating straight on to the wound, and that's what made it sting quite a bit. And me facing this twice a day. I had to go and have my shower; the nurse said it had to be done, so I had no choice. It had to be done; it was for my own good, and I did it.

In situations in which they lacked the knowledge and skills necessary to cure their own illnesses and to relieve their own pain and suffering, patients experienced dependence on others and loss of control. Dependence on others' superior scientific knowledge and technical skills might have been more reassuring had it not also involved repeated experiences of invasive and painful procedures. The experience of *being wounded* made the patients acutely aware of their vulnerability and the need for vigilance in the face of the always present potential for future wounding and harm. What was even more difficult to come to terms with was a deeper and less comprehensible sense of dependence on the benevolence of those who inflicted pain. In a situation in which their bodies had failed them, and in a world that had become unpredictable and often hostile, they needed to believe that those on whom they had to depend would not carelessly or intentionally harm them further. This belief in others' underlying benevolence depended on the procedures being seen as necessary and the ensuing pain as *unavoidable*.

In the context of their situation, patients constructed their experience of inflicted pain as unavoidable and therefore as presenting no other choices but to be endured. If the pain was seen as *punishment* or the reasons behind it questioned, then such perceptions and questions were directed toward some outside source and not toward those inflicting the pain. Even *the good-but nurses,* at whose hands patients experienced more pain than when attended by other nurses, were seen as basically caring and technically capable. Their sensitivity and effectiveness were questioned but not their essential benevolence.

Ultimately, both patients with cancer and those with burn injuries lived with the hope that the painful treatments would help them recover and *become themselves again.* They saw themselves as dependent on others for treatments that would repair their deficient bodies and the inflicted pain as a series of traumatic experiences through which they would have to pass if they were to emerge as intact and whole persons again. Pain was a challenge to be faced with determination and courage, but it was also an overwhelming force that threatened the person's will to live, an embodied sensation unequaled in its immediacy and demand for attention, an experience that left tiredness, exhaustion, and even despair in its wake. Even as different episodes of inflicted pain brought to awareness different meanings of such pain, the questions as to why it had to hurt remained largely unanswered.

However, as Benner and Wrubel (1989) suggest, people do not only constitute their experiences of illness and pain, they are also constituted by them. Bodily pain has the capacity to engage the person, to create a rift between self and body, and to alter the ways in which the person is situated in his or her lifeworld.

BEING CONSTITUTED BY THE EXPERIENCE OF INFLICTED PAIN

Pain is an embodied experience, imposing its presence by its intensity and its spatiality, its location within a particular part of the body. Pain is also an aversive experience that we wish to avoid, so when it is present, it is experienced as something that is at once within the person and at the same time an intruder from which the person wishes to be relieved. It is an alien entity with a power to inhabit the body and to alter it in ways that are unsettling and disturbing to the person. While pain may be both invisible and in large measure unshareable, for the patients in this study, its impact was tangible and sometimes overwhelming. In particular, the experience of inflicted pain changed their sense of themselves as embodied beings and their sense of personal situation, particularly in terms of their experience of *lived space* and *lived time.*

Losing and regaining a sense of embodied self

To have pain, especially inflicted pain, is to have to attend to it and to its impact on the self. The taken-for-granted sense of just being oneself is lost as the person is confronted with the unfamiliar and uncomfortable body that hurts and offers no way to escape. The impact of illness and injury on the embodied self was discussed earlier; in particular, attention was drawn to the significance of patients *feeling different and being different*—of being deconstructed by their suffering and to their almost desperate need to feel that they could *become themselves again.* To the extent that it was possible to separate the impact of pain from the overall impact of illness and treatment on the patients' sense of embodiment, it may be said that pain focused their attention on their embodied being, it underscored their loss of control in the situation, and it helped them to apprehend their experience as one of endurance.

Caught in a situation in which diagnostic and treatment procedures came to be seen as necessary and associated pain as unavoidable, patients became aware of their lived bodies as *exposed, vulnerable, wounded* and *hurting.* They felt keenly their inability to use their habitual, skilled bodies to defend themselves against the pain and to cope with it. Even the "precultural body" (Benner & Wrubel, 1989, p. 70), with its inborn skills of withdrawing from the source of discomfort or pain, could not be allowed to act. Instead, patients had to use deliberate effort to restrain their bodies and their voices. Unable to control outside events and others' actions, they were distressed by the constraints of a situation that placed their bodily needs in opposition to the social norms of the hospital environment. In the following exemplar, the young man illustrates the inner conflict of needing to give external reality and voice to his pain while at the same time feeling constrained to the point of total containment of the pain within the body:

> [On being lowered into a saline bath]…all the excruciating pain, it just shoots through my body. I just want to scream.
>
> (But you don't.)
>
> I am too scared to.
>
> (Why?)

I feel embarrassed. I should [scream]. It's better to let it all out than to hold it in....I just want to scream, but I can't. 'Cause I know I can't. Not in here.

This patient's experience went much deeper than personal embarrassment or social politeness. There was real fear of what screaming would do to his sense of intactness as a person and to the last vestige of control he was trying to retain in the situation. His habitual, skilled body was inadequate for the task, and the conscious, deliberate effort he made could not free him from the pain:

If I try to control myself, it might not hurt as much, and I just can't....I feel I should be able to do something toward it...[tears roll down his face] See, I can lie here now with the pain and just let it subside into me, or else I can do what the nurses do, put my oxygen mask on and take big, deep breaths, but no matter what I do, it's still the same pain I've got.

To the patients themselves, one of the most obvious ways in which they felt they were constituted by pain was in the *tiredness* they felt at the end of and in the periods between painful procedures. They felt *weary*, *tired*, *exhausted*, and *worn out* by the intensity of the pain, the tension and vigilance needed to face and endure it, and by the protracted nature of some of the procedures. The tiredness was unlike any previously known tiredness following physical exertion. In their current situation, they felt a pervasive sense of *weariness* and *energy depletion* and an almost overwhelming need to sleep in order to recoup their strength and be able to face new pain. During protracted procedures, patients became aware of tiredness that lowered their tolerance to discomfort and pain and made even thinking and speech an effort, as in the following exemplar in which the patient is describing a procedure that lasted just over 90 minutes:

After about half an hour or three quarters of an hour of being paced through [a dressing change], I felt I was becoming terribly tired, and I found it almost hard to concentrate on what she [nurse] was saying....I really felt that I just wanted to be left with my head down and being able to close my eyes with nothing being said at all....My tolerance level became a little bit low, and it was just like, "Forget it! I just want the whole thing to be finished" at that stage...[having] to make answers, which took effort...a mental effort...tiring, very tiring.

[Afterward she felt] exhausted....I guess I was physically tired because I had been lying in one position. I was very stiff, and I was very tense. [sighs deeply] And I think also because I was so emotionally upset by the whole thing. I had no trust in the Morphine at all, that it was actually going to ease the pain. It just...it had no impact....I am sorry, but it didn't work at all. I was looking for some kind of relief, but I could not find it at all.

Tiredness was experienced as both energy depletion and as a form of energy reallocation. Coping with pain required energy, and the more energy that was expended on pain, the less there was for anything else. On occasions, patients missed eating their meals or asked that nurses call their families and ask them not to visit because they felt too tired to cope with any other demands. Just coping with pain was all they could deal with at that particular time, with all their energy directed toward keeping pain at bay:

I've got no choice but to sit in here and face this pain. All my energy is going in [to] this pain and that's getting it away from me. I feel that the energy that I used to play tennis is all going into this painful sickness that I have. That's where my energy is going. That's what I feel.

The sense of having no choice, of not being in control, of being caught up in a body and a situation in which the person was not the actor but one acted upon permeated the patients' experience and was difficult to overcome. It was not until most of the wounds had healed and the pain subsided that patients with burn injuries started to feel that they were *becoming themselves again*. At this stage of recovery, the person could face painful procedures through a different body, one that could assume a more confident stance, with less tension and vigilance than previously. To some patients, it came almost as a surprise that their bodies, which had gone through so much pain, could once again be a source of good feelings. The healing was not complete, and the pain remained a possibility with each procedure, but there was also a sense of the embodied person opening out to the world again, with a slowly gathering awareness of strength and confidence. Where pain had meant *wounding, fear, vulnerability*, and *constraint*, its diminution meant a fragile but growing sense of *confidence, strength*, and *openness to others and to the world*. One patient captures this change toward a renewed sense of embodied self in the following interview excerpt:

It's not as bad now, but it is something that I still tense up a little bit about. And I don't say it's something that I look forward to either because the hand to me still looks very, very tender, and there are parts of it which are quite painful. And I think it's hard for the nurse to actually recognize which parts are really sore. But I would say generally, I am much more relaxed at dressing times now.

It was just yesterday, I think, when the girls [nurses] were coming round with the medicines, and I thought to myself for the first time, "Today I can choose whether or not I want any pain killer." And it was really quite a funny feeling...a good feeling. It's a wonderful feeling....I feel stronger in myself...a little bit more trusting of what's going on.

For the patients with cancer, inflicted pain and chemotherapy brought similar experiences of *losing the sense of embodied self,* of feeling *wounded, vulnerable* and no longer in control. However, they found it much more difficult to feel that they were *becoming themselves again* while their treatment continued. Their embodied experience was not of gradual healing but of an ongoing battle being waged within their bodies by the cancer and the drugs with which they were being injected. Thus, inflicted pain was a continuing reminder of their diseased bodies. It not only did not diminish over time, but as the incidence of unsuccessful venepunctures increased, so did the patients' experiences of pain, vulnerability and defenselessness. Their bodies showed all the signs of being sick and impaired as much by the treatment as by the disease, while healing and *becoming themselves again* lay somewhere in the uncertain future. Thus, regaining a sense of embodied self was particularly difficult for patients with cancer, with inflicted pain punctuating their existence and highlighting their lack of autonomy and control.

Losing and regaining a sense of personal situation

We are not only embodied, but through our embodiment, we also inhabit a world by being situated in it. Illness and pain can disturb a person's situatedness, whether this be by the necessity for hospitalization, changes in social relationships and activities, or insecurities and doubts that arise once the familiar, taken-for-granted involvement in the world is challenged. Personal situation is much more than the physical and social environment in which the person lives. It has many facets, and it has many ways of influencing the person and being influenced in return (Benner & Wrubel, 1989). The aspects of the situation that stand out from the experience of patients subjected to inflicted pain are *lived space* and *lived time.*

Pain and *lived space*

To have pain inflicted and be constrained from moving away from the situation influences how the person experiences the space in which he or she must remain. Pain in particular can transform *lived space* of an ordinary room or bed into a place of discomfort and fear, a space that feels hostile and in which the person feels exposed and vulnerable. Patients with cancer were acutely aware of the contrast between the safety and comfort of home and the very different feelings engendered by the laboratory and clinic rooms. These were places to which they *hated having to come*, in which they felt *restricted* to the point of feeling *claustrophobic*. These were also places in which others broke social norms of appropriate bodily distance without seeking patient's permission.

For example, nurses usually sat close to and facing the patient (seated in an armchair) in order to insert the needle and administer intravenous chemotherapy. In this position, nurses' legs touched patients' legs, sometimes being interlocked. While nurses referred to this as "playing knees" and used their own bodies to sense patients' responses during therapy (e.g., tensing or attempting to draw back), patients invariably expressed discomfort with such physical closeness. When hurt by nurses' actions, they had no safety space, no room to draw away. In other situations, such an intrusion into their personal space might have been welcomed, but in this context, it meant the expectation of wounding and pain with no possibility of escape. One patient captured this feeling in vivid terms when he described sitting down in the arm chair "like sitting in an electric chair."

Patients with burn injuries were particularly aware of the places of safety and places where they felt vulnerable and open to wounding and hurt. The treatment room with its large stainless steel bath was the place of dressing changes, saline baths and pain. Their beds, on the other hand, provided the one secure space to which they could retreat. One patient describes her feelings on being returned to her bed after a painful bath and grafting surgery:

> Safe!…Just safe.…Just relieved.…I really didn't want to go anywhere at all. I just wanted to remain in one place, one safe place, and this was it.

There were times, however, when the spatial separation between the place of treatment and place of safety was broken: for example, when the treatment room was being used by others, some patients had to undergo changes of dressings while remaining in their beds. In such situations, the place of safety was transformed into a place of pain, not just for the duration of the procedure, but in a more permanent sense. When revisited, the space in which patients had been hurt previously brought back the experience of the pain and hurt. The body as a knower had learned that particular place was a place of pain, and as Scarry (1985, p. 110) suggests, "what is remembered in the body is well remembered," and a person cannot be compelled to unlearn it. For some patients, even their beds could no longer provide a place of safety.

For the patients hurt by inflicted pain, particular places in which the pain had occurred became places where they not only were not themselves, but they were places in which they experienced the true depth of their alienation and loss of control. Thus, for the patients with cancer, the laboratory and the clinic were *places to which they had to come*, places that were not visited in passing but places one had to talk oneself into visiting, places in which the waiting was profoundly uncomfortable, and places that the person was *eager to leave* as quickly as possible:

> I was grateful that they let me go home for the weekend, but at the same time, I wondered if that slowed the progress of my arm. I didn't know. For my body and myself I felt lovely going home, but on the Monday when they actually took the dressing off after two days, the bandage was quite wet. And I wondered if allowing me to go out like that was a good thing for my arm. For myself, yes. But I'm not sure about the injury, you see, whether it was good for that?...[But it made] such a difference, especially the first time I went home....I don't know what it was. It sort of was like a depression came over me. And then when I went home for the weekend, I came back...I was ready for anything. They could do anything to me.

Home and hospital, treatment rooms and waiting rooms, patients' beds to which they could retreat after painful procedures, all provided different experiences of *lived space* for the patients. Because inflicted pain occurred in a specific place, it influenced the way in which patients felt situated during the weeks or months of their treatment. They developed a sense of situation in which spatiality of pain was not only its embodied characteristic, but also a quality of the space they inhabited for a time. Thus, their personal situation was constituted by pain, both by bringing to awareness the lived reality of space as a context for inflicted pain as well as by sharpening their appreciation for the safety and comfort characterizing lived space in which the person could feel at home.

Pain and *lived time*

People are situated in terms of their lived space and also in terms of their experience of time. Pain can influence the personal experience of time, usually by slowing it down and by extending the period of painfulness. For the patients in this study, initial injury or diagnosis brought an interruption to their *lived time*. The unself-conscious, smooth flow of life was suddenly arrested, and the taken-for-granted future seemed both distant and unclear. Caught in an uncomfortable and often painful present, some patients found it difficult to project themselves into a better future. For a time at least, some simply could not do it. But there was also a more focused way in which inflicted pain altered their immediate sense of temporality, constituting their personal situation into one of sometimes endless pain and of limited endurance that they feared would not last as long as the pain.

For some patients with burn injuries, the initial pain was so severe that they felt overwhelmed not only by its intensity, but also by its apparent endlessness. Others became aware of pain's interminable quality when instead of easing off following their evening change of dressings the pain would persist, making it impossible for them to sleep. A restless night of wakefulness and pain, followed by painful procedures when day-time arrived, left patients feeling exhausted and in constant pain.

Episodes of extremely intense pain inflicted during dressing changes had a particularly profound effect on the patients' experience of time. The following exemplar captures one patient's experience of pain, which he rated at 9.99 on a 10-point scale:

> It probably lasted only 4 or 5 minutes that particular instance, but to me it seemed an awful lot longer. I even had the feeling that the nurses were moving slowly....I know they weren't, but everything just slowed down because that was hurting so much and relief wasn't coming soon enough. So I think a second turns into a minute and a minute into an hour.

The combination of painfulness, tiredness, and time that moved slowly was common in situations of extensive dressing changes. More frequently, it occurred when nurses decided to perform the procedure in stages, taking time out in between to attend to other duties:

> I wasn't particularly looking forward to the dressing....I wasn't looking forward to looking at the hand, and I didn't think the pain would be as severe as it was. It took *so long*. I think that was one of the hardest

things for me because it took so long....It took 4 hours, and that was such a big strain on the system. Because it was so bad I asked one of the nurses to make a call to my mother to say I am not wanting her to come in. I didn't really want to see visitors at all. I just felt so tired and so shaken by the whole thing.

(What do you think shook you?)

The pain! My tolerance level for the pain has normally been quite good, but yesterday it was bad....She [nurse] would work for half an hour, and then she would leave. She would leave me for about half an hour to an hour. And then she would come back, and she would work for another half hour, and then she would go off again. And I found that distressing. I found that even worse because it lengthened the whole process unnecessarily. The thing that I wanted her to do was to just get the whole thing over and done with, wrapped up.

The difficulties that patients had in coping with such extended procedures related mainly to their experience of time and its quality. The intervals when the patient was left alone were not times of safety or times of comfort since the patient still felt exposed and vulnerable, with more pain to come. The whole procedure was prolonged, and the time when the person could retreat into a place of safety was delayed. Thus, the patient needed to be *wrapped up* in order to feel less vulnerable and, at least until the next dressing change, protected from further pain infliction.

For the patients with cancer, the time in pain was relatively brief, with needle insertion (when successful on first attempt) taking only a second or two. As the incidence of unsuccessful venepunctures increased, however, this time of pain became the focal point of the experience of having intravenous chemotherapy. The waiting time in the Laboratory and the Oncology Clinic became a *time of anticipation* and concern with how many attempts at venepuncture would need to be made and how much they would hurt. The time of chemotherapy administration, lasting from a few minutes to half an hour, also had a quality of anticipation as well as vigilance about it and went very slowly. Patients' main concern during this time was the possibility of a *burning* or *painful sensation,* which would signal seepage of drugs out of the vein being injected and the need for reinsertion of the needle and, thus, further pain.

Patients with cancer who accepted the offer to wear "the cold cap" in the attempt to prevent hair loss provided another example of *lived time.* They experienced not only the discomfort and pain of having the head wrapped in icy-cold cloth, but also the extended time needed for chemotherapy when this procedure was employed. The "clock time" of an extra 30 to 40 minutes the patient spent in the treatment chair was further extended by the subjective perception of *time moving very slowly* in this situation. Eventually, when despite this particularly uncomfortable measure patients started to lose hair, they invariably expressed a sense of relief since the "cold-cap" treatment could be abandoned and the "chemo time" reduced.

The anticipatory time during which patients remembered past pain and tried to anticipate what would happen in the immediate future often went just as slowly as the time in pain. It made them aware of being impatient, restless, and uncomfortable in the situation and of wanting *time to speed up* so that the treatment would be over and they could leave their present place and time.

For the patients in this study, there was a time of waiting, a time of anticipation, a time of unease and discomfort, a time of pain, a time of relief and safety, a time of looking to the future, and a time of feeling caught in the present. These were all aspects of *lived time*, time that was personal, moving at different speeds, and situating the person in a different lifeworld.

Endurance of pain involves being bodily in the situation and at the same time not becoming overwhelmed by it. It also involves constituting the experience and finding meaning within the situation. When isolated from its context, inflicted pain has no purpose and makes no sense to the experiencing person. The pain and the enduring of it need to be constituted into something that has meaning and purpose. In other contexts, clinically inflicted pain my hold other meanings, but for the patients who participated in this study, the inflicted pain was such an integral part of their situation that they grasped it as essentially unavoidable. The procedures through which it was generated were accepted as necessary, but the pain itself was simply there, real, immediate and unavoidable.

The experience of nurses, as those who inflict pain in the course of their work, who have their own perceptions of pain which they help to generate, and their own ways of coping with the outcomes of their actions, is discussed in the next chapter.

Chapter 6
Inflicting And Relieving Pain:
The Lifeworld Of Nursing Practice

Throughout this study, particular attention has been given to the context of the lived experience of clinically inflicted pain. Inflicted pain is unique in the extent to which it merges subject and context. Nurses, normally an element of the patient's situation, become the ones who control the cause of the pain—its onset, continuation and termination. Yet at the same time, whether or not they wish it, they are excluded from entering into a direct experience of that pain. Despite their physical closeness and the sharing in the tactile encounter during which pain is generated, patients and nurses inhabit different lifeworlds and so apprehend inflicted pain from very different perspectives. Phenomenology stresses the inherent uniqueness in how people experience their own bodies, which is different from how they experience external objects, including others' bodies. In the words of Scarry (1985, p. 13), "To have pain is to have *certainty*, to hear about pain is to have *doubt*." The worlds of patients and nurses are separated by a gulf of embodied experience, yet they are also inextricably linked.

NURSES' EMBODIED EXPERIENCE OF PAINFUL PROCEDURES

Inflicted pain can alter a patient's sense of embodiment and being-in-the-world. Such alterations can be profound and longlasting. Nurses, however, cannot physically experience the pain they are inflicting nor its impact on the embodied self since it is not their bodies that are handed over, wounded, hurt, or restrained in their expression. Indeed, it is **because** they feel no pain that nurses are able to perform procedures that patients experience as painful and can work in settings where pain infliction is a common part of work. Yet if the patients' experiences of pain were totally private and inaccessible to nurses, then infliction of pain would not be a problem or a source of stress for nurses. If they were unaware of patients' suffering, then they would not feel a need to shield themselves from it. It is because they **did** sense something of the patient's experience, because they *grasped the situation* (Benner & Wrubel, 1989, p. 49) in a direct way as one of pain for the patient that nurses in this study reported a sense of dis-ease in their own being. In their own terms, nurses found pain infliction *stressful*, while at the same time, they found a great deal of satisfaction in the performance of the procedures that were the source of pain for the patient. This paradoxical situation provided the framework for the nurses' lived experience of inflicting pain.

The stress and the satisfaction in nurses' work

In this study, while nurses said their work was *stressful*, they chose to work in the Burn Care Unit and generally had no plans to move into another field of nursing. As discussed in Appendix A, the Unit had a very stable nursing workforce, with an average of 3.6 years practice in that setting. Of the 15 nurses who took part in the study, all but two had worked there for at least 18 months, and all but one intended to continue working in the Unit. What was the attraction? The nurses provided two answers to this question.

First, the work in the Burn Care Unit was varied, interesting and challenging. The nurses said there were several positive aspects to the work in the Burn Care Unit: for example, the Unit catered to patients of all ages, from young infants to the very old; it included general plastic surgery as well as burn cases; and the majority of patients recovered. Both registered and enrolled nurses felt that they were given genuine responsibility and were trusted to make judgements in relation to patient care. There was little in the work that was routine or boring.

Second, and more important, nurses came to, and chose to stay in, the Burn Care Unit because they enjoyed the technical aspects of their work. Unlike their experience in other fields of nursing, here they felt that both the underlying disease process and the treatment involving people with burns were directly visible. The initial damage could be extensive, but each step of the healing process, each grafting procedure, each piece of healed skin could be seen and the success credited to the nurses' skill and technical expertise.

Individual nurses felt a commitment to a particular patch of skin they had been the first to uncover after grafting or had added later to a part of a graft that had initially failed to take. They described feeling quite possessive about such patches of skin, treating them with particular care and resenting anyone else touching them. This type of objectification of the patient could lead to some rather uneasy exchanges between nurses and patients when, as in the following case, patients responded with black humour:

[As the nurse pulled the dressing away from the wound, the patient inhaled deeply and loudly, and then held his breath.]

Nurse: "Oh, I am glad that's painful. That's good. It's not as deep as I thought it looked. It's a bit hard to tell, especially with the [silver sulphadiazine] cream. It looked a bit white here, but it's only cream."

Patient: [forcing a nervous laugh] "I am glad it's sore for you!"

[The nurse then went on to explain how interested nurses usually are in particular patches of skin they had helped to heal or graft.]

Nurse: "I'll often ask the patient how 'my' skin is doing because I would have been the one who applied it."

Patient: "I wouldn't mind, so long as you remember that I am quite attached to it myself!"

The above exemplar captures not only the objectification of the patient's body into patches that have healed and those that have not, it also shows the instrumental value of pain for the nurse. To her, pain was not *hurting* or *wounding*, as it might have been to the patient; rather, it was a helpful sign of the limited tissue damage: the burn injury was not so deep as to have destroyed peripheral nerve endings, and that was something "good," something to be glad about. In this situation, pain was the confirmation of the healing the nurse's actions had helped to produce and, therefore, a source of satisfaction. Rather than responding to the lived experience of the patient, the nurse's concern was with the meaning the pain had for her.

The difficult and quite intricate dressings that often occupied the main part of the nurses' working day came through very strongly as a reason why they enjoyed their work. Such procedures provided technical variety and challenge and served as important sources of satisfaction for the nurse. The following examples were typical of the nurses' responses to the question of why they chose to work and go on working in the Burn Care Unit:

> I asked to come here because I just felt I was not learning enough new things in the surgical wards. I had reached stalemate. I wanted something more exciting to do, and I had a bent towards big dressings and just a little bit more technical nursing than what I had been doing.

> I like to do dressings. I like to do intricate things, I enjoy it. I enjoy laying skin. I like taking tricky stitches out. I enjoy that kind of thing, and I wouldn't get it in any other area.

It was rather paradoxical then that it was the patients' responses to these same technical procedures that provided the main source of stress identified by all the nurses as the biggest drawback to working in the Burn Care Unit. Low staff numbers, a problem in other parts of the hospital, was not an issue in the Unit. The physical facilities were relatively new, the nursing team supportive, and the medical team approachable and appreciative of the nurses' contribution to patient care. Despite these positive attributes of their work environment, nurses described dressing changes and related procedures as *stressful, emotionally demanding,* and at times *frustrating.* It was less the stress of having to hurt patients and more how the patients responded to being hurt that was the predominant theme in the nurses' descriptions of the negative side of their work.

When patients tolerated painful procedures without overt displays of distress, they were perceived not only as cooperative, but also as *coping.* Nurses felt at ease in such situations, able to concentrate on the technical aspects of the task at hand, and free to complete the procedure at their own pace. At other times, when patients became distressed and indicated that they had difficulties dealing with pain and discomfort, the nurses felt under pressure to either compromise the quality of their technical performance or ignore a patient's distress in order to ensure a thorough job. They came away from such situations feeling *uptight, not nice, mean,* or *cruel,* all the ways of being-in-the-world they felt were forced on them by the patient's behavior.

Generally, adult patients were expected to endure considerable pain without crying, screaming, or becoming uncooperative. Children, however, could not be expected to show the same forbearance and stoicism, and the burden of coping was therefore placed more fully on the nurses, who had to learn how to deal with a child who started crying at the sight of a nurse's uniform and was likely to cry, scream, and lash out during the procedure.

Their greater capacity for self-control meant that adults were expected to minimize behavioral expressions of pain and distress. At the same time, nurses used explanations and verbal reinforcement to encourage stoical behavior in adults. In such situations, nurses could retain considerable emotional distance between themselves and the patient's lived experience. Children, on the other hand, were seen to lack both the capacity for self-control and for reasoning in situations that they perceived as painful and threatening. Their uninhibited responses to painful procedures were the main source of stress for the nurses in the Unit, making them feel *tense, dissatisfied* with the day's work, and drawn further into the patient's experience than they would have preferred. In other words, children's uncontrolled expressions of pain and distress had the power to confront nurses with the impact of their actions and to alter their embodied experience of being involved in the generation of pain. In particular, the child's unrestrained use of his or her body and voice interfered with the nurse's use of their own bodies (to accomplish the task) and voice (to persuade the child of the necessity of the procedure and to elicit quiet cooperation):

> I find it very stressful dealing with burnt children because you can't explain to them as to why you've got to do it....They see a green uniform when you walk in, and they turn the other way....You can't say, "Well, you really need your dressing changed." They don't care. All they know is that you are hurting them.

> They see you coming, they know it's time for a dressing, they open their mouths and they don't stop until you wheel them back into their room. And whether it's going to hurt or not...they will still scream at the thought of it. And that I find hard. You have to just block it out almost and just get on with what you were going to do.

> As soon as you start inflicting pain on a child, that's all they will remember. And I don't think that they realize as time goes on that they are better. The fact is, you are doing the dressing and it hurts, regardless of whether or not they are just about fully healed. They will still react just like they did in the beginning....I can remember two of them that literally had to be dragged along the floor just to get them to the bathroom [where treatments are carried out]. And I mean that's terror for them....We have to do it because it speeds up healing, cuts down the chances of infection, minimizes their hospital stay, and all that sort of thing. There are a lot of reasons, but it's very difficult.

It is significant that even though the study dealt only with adults all the nurses spontaneously brought up the subject of children and the stress of having to work on them. Nurses' perceptions of children as unable to appreciate the good intentions of staff or to control their fears and emotional expressions were relevant for two reasons. First, adult patients were contrasted with children and the point made that because they were not children adults could be expected to respond to reasoning, information and verbal reassurance. Thus, nurses expected adult patients to show composure, self-control and, above all, cooperation, regardless of how painful the procedure or how much or little pain relief may have been provided. Second, the small number of adult patients who failed to live up to such expectations were considered to be in some way immature and, like children, beyond help by reasoning or other rational means:

> As I said, some people cope very well, they are very willing to please, and they are very cooperative. Those people you don't have a lot of trouble with. It's the person whose pain threshold is low, who may be a bit nervy in his life anyway....You see, over the years I've come to realize that sometimes no amount of talking, no amount of explaining...if a person's got a certain level of fear inside them, you can't resolve it.

> It's not often that you get someone that can't cope. I mean, there's more that cope than can't cope.

Overall, nurses disliked inflicting pain and hurting patients in the process of treatment. Some speculated as to why a way had not been found to treat burn trauma without causing further pain and distress. Pain control approaches such as general anaesthesia, inhalation analgesia, patient-controlled analgesia, and even continuous intravenous infusion of Morphine or other narcotics were usually dismissed as impractical or involving too much risk for the patient. Therefore, nurses considered that inflicting some pain was an inevitable part of their work, which new nurses had to accept and learn to carry out without being overwhelmed by patients' responses. In the following exemplar, a nurse with only 5 months experience in the Burn Care Unit describes her feelings about performing procedures that are painful for the patient and then contrasts her responses with how she sees more experienced nurses approaching their work:

> I find that even after being here 5 months I tend to rationalize a lot of things, like the pain. I particularly found that the really hard thing to

cope with when I first came here was the pain the patients were experiencing. And I used to think, "Why can't I do something to stop this pain, why can't I give them an injection?"...It was really hard to get into thinking, "This person is in pain, okay, fine. He'll be uncomfortable for the next 20 minutes while I do the dressing, but then he'll be all right."...I don't like to cope with that myself, that I am inflicting pain so to speak, but I prepare myself by thinking, "I'll get in there, I'll do it," and in some cases detach yourself from the person for a time, while it hurts.

(How do you manage to do that? How do you achieve that detachment?)

I have to make a conscious effort to stop myself thinking "Oh look, you are hurting so and so." I spend most of my time saying, "I am really sorry. I don't mean to hurt you." And I mean it. I am very sincere about it, but sometimes I have to think, "Okay, this person is in pain, but I have to go ahead and do it."...I just have to make a conscious decision to think, "Get on with it!"

The nurses who have been here [longer] are not hard, but their approach is different to mine. I've heard patients say, "Nurse so and so, she's really rough." It's not that they are rough, it's just that they can cope with the pain that the patient is undergoing at the time and just go ahead and do it and not blink an eyelid, whereas I go in there and think, "Oh no, they are in pain. I'll take my time," and supposedly be more gentle....I can be more gentle and not get rid of all the air pockets [under a new graft] whereas they could be so-called "rough," get in there, clean it out, and be doing a thorough job, a better job than me....I sometimes feel very inadequate.

This extract encapsulates several other key issues that exemplify nursing practice and attitudes to the care of patients with burns, which will be discussed later in this chapter. There are several major factors that help to describe nurses' experience of being the ones who inflict pain and go on inflicting it: learning to accept the inevitability of pain rather than questioning its necessity in specific situations; learning to see pain as temporary and therefore of less consequence; learning to rationalize about pain and teach oneself not to pay attention to it; learning to think that a nurse is coping with patients' pain when he/she is able to ignore signs of pain and distress; and learning that technical performance counts more than the amount of pain inflicted or avoided. The exemplar also captures something of the ethos of the Burn Care Unit, that is, the expectation that patients will endure their pain and be cooperative and that nurses will ensure that regardless of how much pain their actions may cause technical procedures will be done and will be done thoroughly.

Oncology Clinic nurses

Nurses in the Oncology Clinic expressed their work experience rather differently. First, they had chosen to work in the clinic for a variety of reasons, none of which had to do with the technical procedures. They administered chemotherapy on only one day per week, and they liked the change from work in other outpatient clinics or departments and the regular hours and free weekends. The workload was generally lighter than elsewhere, and nurses were able to get to know the patients over the months of their therapy.

Second, performing procedures that were potentially or actually painful to patients was not something that these nurses found particularly stressful, nor did it concern them to the point that they wished to change it in any way. Their work was demanding, with three of the four clinic nurses planning to look for a different field of practice, but their reasons had nothing to do with pain infliction. The situations these nurses found particularly stressful were those related to *having to communicate with patients whose prognosis was frequently very poor, having to administer chemotherapy when its benefits were uncertain,* and *having to deal with "difficult" patients* whose initial anxiety did not abate and who were perceived as *not coping well* with the impact of chemotherapy:

It is stressful because you know that they are possibly going to die from the disease that they have. And it's hard to talk about it; it's hard to get the patients to get around to talking about it together. Often they don't want to, and I find that really hard. I find I have to work really hard at what I say. That's probably the most stressful part of it....Even Mrs H, her awful wound, that doesn't distress me so much. I can accept that because I've seen that probably lots of times before. The thing that distresses me is that she thinks it is going to get better....Who is going to tell her it's not going to get better?

Although Oncology Clinic nurses did not consider venepunctures and the intravenous administration of chemotherapy to be painful, they did recognize that patients became anxious and distressed when the procedure was unsuccessful and had to be repeated. Each nurse was concerned not to be the one who caused local tissue damage and made the job more difficult for the next person. For these reasons, rather than because they recognized that their actions caused pain to the patient, nurses usually gave up after two unsuccessful attempts and asked a physician to insert the intravenous needle. Asked to comment on how much pain she expected patients to tolerate in the course of intravenous chemotherapy, one nurse responded,

> I hope never to find that out. I hope to get one [needle into the vein] before they run out of tolerance, without subjecting them to too much. I think that they become increasingly tense. Well, it's unpleasant for one thing....I always find it difficult. "How long do you keep trying before you get someone else to have a go?" It's not really on past two [attempts], is it? Well, that's what I think....Should you be so confident in your ability to get one that you keep trying?...To my mind that's not a great idea. Because you still might not get it after the third, or fourth, or fifth go, so then you have to go and get someone else. By that time you've filled them full of holes and puckerooed [shattered] chances for the next person....So that's my philosophy, if you can't get it in twice, then get someone else.

These nurses were also extremely vigilant with chemotherapy administration, making sure that there was no leakage or spillage of the cytotoxic solution. The awareness that the resulting tissue damage could be extensive and that the nurse's reputation might suffer as the result was evident, but once again, there was no indication that the resulting pain for the patient was a significant concern:

> My main concern is "will it affect their arm, their veins?"...I've heard stories of great big sloughing ulcers and things like that from chemotherapy. That would be my major concern. I would hate to do that to somebody. I would hate to be the person that would be branded with having done that to them. That would be my fault.

Thus, for the nurses in the Oncology Clinic, neither the satisfaction nor the stress experienced in their work had any direct connection to the performance of what patients experienced as painful procedures. Rather, their satisfaction came from working conditions that had little to do with patients, and their stress came from being part of medical therapy that far too often in their experience proved damaging or ineffective.

Before considering the strategies that nurses in the Burn Care Unit used to cope with the paradox of stress and satisfaction in their work, it is necessary to present nurses' perceptions of inflicted pain and its relief.

NURSES' PERCEPTIONS OF INFLICTED PAIN

If there was a paradox in what Burn Care Unit nurses considered to be the source of both stress and satisfaction in their work, there was also a paradox in how they perceived the pain generated through their work. Despite the visibility of patients' wounds and the directness of nurses' physical actions when providing wound care, many instances of patients' pain were not recognized, named, or acknowledged as pain. Pain could be qualified, defined, explained, or denied in such a way that it often became *invisible* and *not real*. Yet, overall, inflicted pain was difficult to ignore, and it was perceived and presented to patients as largely *inevitable* and thus inescapably *real* as well as *nonharmful* and, by some nurses, even as *beneficial*. This paradoxical perception in turn resulted in both denial of pain in some instances and its interpretation as inevitable but of no great concern in many others.

Visible and invisible pain

By definition all pain is invisible; it is a private experience that a person not in pain cannot know directly. Yet relief of pain and suffering depends on a private experience being shared to the extent that a person's pain becomes another's concern and thus acquires visibility and a social dimension. Making pain visible requires that it be given voice, not only by the person in pain, but also by those with the power to relieve it. Thus, making pain visible is a joint project which requires that the patient's body and voice are believed rather than being doubted or by-passed (Scarry, 1985). There are in clinical practice, however, many ways of keeping pain private and invisible and thus denying or casting doubt on its reality.

One way of recognizing the reality of pain and making it visible is to anticipate it and prepare the patient adequately for it. In the Burn Care Unit, this happened when nurses acknowledged that certain circumstances would result in pain and acted accordingly. For example, pain was more likely to be anticipated in relation to the first saline bath, debridement, first change of dressings after skin grafting, or on premature removal of donor site dressings. In such situations, nurses were more likely to recognize the potential for pain, to provide some pain-relieving medication beforehand and to acknowledge patients' pain openly, sometimes apologizing or expressing regrets about actions that might have contributed to a patient's pain. The following extract from a nurse's interview shows the reasoning and anticipation used with a particular patient:

I decided to give him intravenous Morphine for his dressing to his hand because it is his first dressing. Because, based on past experiences, first dressings can be very painful, and intravenous Morphine works much, much better than IM [intramuscular] Morphine, much faster, and it just seems to control the pain so much better. It's not always practical because we don't always have a doctor available to give it, but if there is a doctor in the ward, I don't see any reason why not to do it....Where you've had the skin laid it isn't going to be that painful. It's where there is no skin and you clean it and try to get off any debris, that is going to hurt. I think the object of a dressing is to get it done as swiftly and as efficiently as you can, and that's what I tried to do.

He might need IM pain relief tomorrow because he is having a big dressing off his leg and his hand. It should get significantly less and less painful. The first dressing is always the worst after a graft, mainly because it is so hideously stuck....If you take the donor area [dressing] right down, it's fiendish.

On the other hand, there were many reasons given as to why patients should not experience pain, despite their injuries and the potentially wounding procedures performed on them. *Deep* burns (third-degree) were not expected to be painful, either at rest or during dressing changes, even though the patients' experience did not support this view. Furthermore, opioids such as Morphine were expected to not just reduce, but eliminate both procedural and residual pain. Again, this was not borne out in the patients' experience. As their burn injuries began to heal, patients were expected to experience less (and tolerate more) pain, not only at rest, but also during dressing changes, and as one nurse expressed it, they should be able to "cope with just about anything done to them."

The normative approach nurses usually adopted toward pain led to constant comparisons being made between different patients, the relative severity of their injuries, and the acceptability of behaviors manifested as the result of inflicted pain. Nurses also weighed specific instances of pain against factors that would either justify the apparent severity and impact of pain or provide reasons why the particular pain should not be regarded with concern. Thus, a distinction was frequently made between *real pain* and other uncomfortable and unpleasant sensations that were not defined as pain:

I feel the only *real* pain that she had was when I took the stitches out; she had very real pain then. I also felt there was a little bit of pain following on the inside of her calf around the edges of the graft because it is quite superficial, and quite often taking that paranet [paraffin impregnated dressing] off it does sting, so there would have been pain then. But it would not have been great, it just would have been an instant thing....She did have a little cry....I think it was just a sort of built-up emotion. But other than that, I don't think there was any real pain.

Different forms of patient behavior were also taken as indications that the pain was either absent or minimal. When they refrained from vocal expressions such as groaning, crying or screaming or did not *complain* about pain, nurses took that as an indication that patients experienced little or no pain. When, on the other hand, patients did provide vocal or other indications of pain, nurses frequently defined these as signs of *anxiety, fear* or even *hysteria* rather than pain. In situations where children or young adolescents gave vocal and free expression to their pain, some nurses commented that it was the nurses rather than the patients who needed Valium™ or loud music from the radio as a way of coping with the stress. At times, there was even a suggestion that if the nurse could cope with the patient's behavior, then either there was no pain or the pain was at an acceptable level and did not require relief.

The following excerpt refers to a patient who was admitted with 12 percent, mainly first- and second-degree, burns. The nurse was describing his first saline bath and debridement on the day of his admission to hospital. His only analgesic medication was an intramuscular injection of Pethidine™ given more than 4 hours earlier:[1]

Well, I wasn't feeling a great deal then because he is only a superficial burn. If he was not under any sort of pain control, I wouldn't have gone ahead with it because I can't do anything to a patient unless they are sedated or painfree. Because it's just...it's awful watching someone in pain. So it's better for *me* to have them out of pain, and it's also better for *them* because they are more cooperative....I decided that a shower was in order, and he wasn't so badly burnt that he couldn't tolerate a shower, and he was capable of walking because it's only from the chest area up. I could see he was a nice, pleasant man as well; he wasn't obnoxious. So I assessed all that....He only had a couple of lesions that needed debriding, so I knew that wouldn't be painful, and I would have stopped if there had been any pain...but I felt completely fine. It wasn't traumatic at all in any way.

The patient's experience was, however, rather different. Unable to see because of facial burns and swelling, this man insisted that his wife be allowed to stay with him during this initial treatment:

It felt sore...really strange because I couldn't see. That's the worst part of it....It's hard when you can't see when something's happening to you...in pain at the same time, the burns all heating up and hurting.

(How much did it hurt?)

About 7 [on a 10-point scale], more pain than when the accident happened.

When, as in the above example, the nurse made decisions without validating her assessment with the patient, then the pain could be made invisible. The patient's restraint of his body and voice and the nurse's focus on her own rather than the patient's emotional response allowed the nurse to feel satisfied with her performance while failing to establish what the experience was like for the patient. Lack of sharing and consultation with the patients, discussed more fully later in this chapter, was one important factor that made possible the apparent invisibility of pain and allowed nurses to retain distance between their actions and patients' experiences.

The first step in this alleviation of pain is not to doubt its reality but to acknowledge its presence. To doubt the reality of patients' pain or dismiss it as merely something unpleasant or uncomfortable "amplifies the suffering of those already in pain" (Scarry, 1985, p. 7). It also creates distance between the patient and the nurse, making understanding of the patient's experience of pain more difficult and its alleviation less likely. In the midst of inflicted pain, adult patients usually try to be cooperative and to retain composure, and they do it by restraining the body and the voice. Thus, the already private experience is made even less visible to others. It is when nurses accept such controlled outward expression as the whole of the patient's experience that pain becomes invisible and, therefore, easier for nurses to ignore and overlook.

Inevitable pain

The nature of patients' injuries and the procedures performed on them in the Burn Care Unit meant that not all pain could be treated as invisible. A young man who screamed during his first saline bath, a woman who cried and shook uncontrollably while her hand was being debrided, and a man who cried when he remembered a particularly painful episode, all gave forceful evidence of severe and overwhelming pain. To be able to continue working in this setting, nurses needed to learn to cope with such overt expressions of pain. Strong influences on how they should view patients' pain and how they might cope with it came from the group values and norms impressed on new staff members. The working ethos of the unit was that much of the inflicted pain was *inevitable* and that except in extreme cases, when general anaesthesia might be given, both nurses and patients had to accept such pain as an *expected part of the process of recovery* and as something to be approached with fortitude and the will to endure. In the words of one senior nurse,

I think we all know in nursing...any sort of nursing, there are procedures that are carried out on patients that are unpleasant. We know they are going to cause a certain amount of discomfort before you even start....It's something that has to be done. I don't ever feel good about it. I think it's something we all have to prepare ourselves for. In fact, before I do a huge, a large burn dressing...I think you have to prepare yourself mentally....I don't think apart from giving general anaesthetic every time you did a procedure that you can make it totally not painful. And I think that's something that you have to accept, and the patient has to accept.

And that's one of the reasons I am not terribly keen on things like Morphine infusions because what I find with Morphine infusions a great deal of the time, the patient stays confused and sometimes agitated and disorientated...and they are not really, what I would call, facing up to or coping with what in this area often has to continue for a great deal of time [i.e., painful procedures].

The nurse in this situation believed that opioids, particularly when administered at more than infrequent and irregular intervals, made patients sleepy and uncooperative and were therefore unhelpful and should be discontinued as soon as possible. At the same time, she reasoned that the pain would recur with each new grafting operation and subsequent dressings and would probably go on for some time. Unless patients were to be allowed to run the risk of drug addiction, they would eventually have to cope with pain without the aid of opioid medication. Since they would eventually have to cope without the aid of strong analgesics, then the sooner they were able to do that, the better. This is what the nurses and, through them, the patients were expected to accept, and the acceptance was defined as *coping with the reality* of burn trauma.

While some nurses who had worked in other burn care units expressed preference for more rigorous approaches to pain management, such as the use of a combination of intravenous Morphine and Valium™, they accepted that such practices were not used in this unit and followed the accepted routines. Given the general expectation that patients would accept their pain as inevitable, it was perhaps not surprising that patients who were seen as *relying on medication* (particularly opioids) to endure the painful procedures performed on them were seen as *not coping,* as in the following extract:

See, [patient] had a Morphine infusion until he came here, and in many ways, I am not sure whether that's done him a service or not.

(In what way?)

Because I feel he doesn't cope with pain at all well at the moment. He certainly is someone I would say isn't coping. His burns...on the top half of his back aren't that deep. So they will be very, very sore. The area where to me they look to be the deepest, and we are told that there shouldn't be a great deal of pain, he is actually complaining and saying it's the most painful....I am not saying that it isn't, but it's just quite an interesting thing.

(What are you using as indication that he is not coping well?)

His requests for pain relief, his obvious distress, obvious physical distress, and just his communication, his whole attitude, he is not eating very well yet, those sorts of things....I think he is at the stage now [8 days after injury] where we have to be firm with him, talk to him, try to talk him through [painful procedures, without use of opioids], make him more comfortable in other ways. Try and alleviate pain by sitting him differently, changing his position, and getting him to eat his lunch, and try and think of something else.

While changes of body position or distraction through brief verbal exchanges with nurses were helpful in dealing with some discomforts and less severe background pain, on their own they were quite inadequate during many episodes of inflicted pain. Inflicted pain was thus not only perceived as inevitable, but in many instances became inevitable.

Nurses' perception of inflicted pain as *inevitable* bestowed a form of reality on it—it happened, and it happened within certain space and time. However, the reality of such pain did not necessarily involve the patient's lived experience. It could be, and often was, defined on the basis of the nurses' experience of dealing with the patient's overt expression of pain. This movement from the patient's lived certainty of pain to the less solid ground of interpretation of changing behaviors may explain some of the disparity between patients' and nurses' accounts of inflicted pain.

As described earlier, patients were very sensitive to the quality of the tactile encounter with nurses during painful procedures and, therefore, to the conditional nature of pain. They accepted some pain as inevitable, but they were also acutely aware of the extent to which inflicted pain could be ameliorated or intensified by particular nurses' actions. Nurses, on the other hand, tended to see the inevitability of pain as an absolute and themselves as lacking the power to alter the experience of pain, as expressed in the following exemplar:

> You could spend an hour and it's still going to be as painful as what you could do something in 5 minutes. You always are as gentle as you can be…and just get them to bear with you. Really…I don't feel even sad. Well, you do, but you just know that it's the best thing for them, and you know it will only take a week or…sometimes it's just the first dressing, and you know it's going to get better. You can get quite hard to it really. Put on a steel face and just do it.…I think you just get used to it.…You get immune to it, and you just face up [to it] and away you go!

When nurses perceived everything about inflicted pain as inevitable, they also perceived themselves as unable to change the situation for the better. Rather than seeing themselves as the ones with the knowledge, resources, and the power to relieve and manage pain, nurses often felt helpless and immobilized in the face of pain they had inflicted. Furthermore, the perception of pain as inevitable absolved nurses from responsibility for its causation. With few exceptions, they felt unable to prevent pain and tried to interpret it as an experience with which the majority of patients could *cope*, that is, endure it with composure and in a way that did not interfere with nurses' work. At the same time, they interpreted pain as nonharmful and even as somehow beneficial to the patient.

Nonharmful and beneficial pain

The difficulty for nurses in the Burn Care Unit was that their daily involvement with patients in pain continually challenged their attempts to make pain *invisible*. And the perception of inflicted pain as *inevitable* did not solve the issue either. They were still faced with the need to act on the patient's body in a way that they knew caused pain to the patient and a sense of *unease* and *stress* to themselves. Because treatment procedures were seldom accomplished without pain, nurses faced a continuing need to justify its infliction, both to the patients and to themselves. Some tried to rationalize pain infliction as something that had to be done and about which there were no choices. In doing so they had to block or overcome their embodied knowledge of pain as something hurtful and wounding and construct it into something *necessary, nonharmful,* and *justified*.

When describing inflicted pain, therefore, nurses did not speak of it as intrinsically bad or as harmful in its consequences. None of the nurses mentioned, at any stage, that having to endure pain was in any way harmful to patients, either as people on whom pain might have a negative impact or in any specific way, whether physiologically or psychologically. Having pain was seen as an expected and inevitable part of recovery. This acknowledgment of the reality of pain was easier to accept when the pain they inflicted was interpreted by nurses as *temporary*, intense only for *brief* periods, and *not taxing* the limits of the patient's endurance:

A little bit [of debridement] doesn't hurt here and there, and that was only a little bit, so I wasn't worried....She is a good patient really....Outwardly she seems to tolerate the dressing and the shower and everything well. She doesn't seem to be in a lot of pain....I would say she would have sort of moderate pain, but I don't think it would last too long or be too severe.

Inflicted pain was also more acceptable to nurses when they perceived that it was *not harmful in the long-term* and *necessary* for patients' recovery. While some nurses talked in general terms about the benefits of treatment procedures (which had the unfortunate effect of also causing some pain), others were quite specific in describing pain itself as *beneficial* rather than harmful. In either case, such interpretations made inflicted pain not only easier to justify to patients, but also more tolerable to nurses:

I didn't like it [inflicting pain] when I first started here...but I am much better now. I guess it's by having been here a while and seen so much and done so many [procedures]. You know that most of the time they are going to be OK. You don't like having to do it, but it's just something that in the end you've got to do. In the long run they are going to benefit from it.

I don't like to inflict pain on people. And I find it quite hard when someone is obviously in a lot of pain. But I've found working here...I know it sounds pretty cruel but...I compensate for inflicting pain on someone by sort of rationalizing and saying that pain will actually help them get better in the long run.

The interpretation of inflicted pain as *temporary*, as *necessary*, and as *not harmful* and possibly even *beneficial* to patients' recovery was an important means by which such pain was made more acceptable and tolerable to nurses. In turn, nurses tried to use this same reasoning to appeal to patients in order to lessen their anxiety and to gain their cooperation. This process of reconstructing pain into a more acceptable form helped to secure patients' cooperation as well as allowing nurses to feel a sense of satisfaction in their work. They could inflict pain and yet at the end of the day feel good about their contribution to patients' healing.

Oncology Clinic nurses

The small amount of tissue damage involved in the performance of venepunctures, especially when contrasted with the systemic effects of chemotherapy, led the Oncology Clinic nurses to conclude that patients experienced little in the way of inflicted pain. They described the waiting for treatment as *difficult* and even *painful* and experiences of nausea and vomiting as *upsetting patients more than pain*. At the same time, there was a tendency to minimize the impact of inflicted pain and to see it as largely unproblematic, as in the following extracts:

I would say it is a small issue. Actual pain, the pain of a needle [being] put in, not many people talk about the pain at all, no....I wonder what I could do? I mean, as I said, I think it's only a small amount of pain.

The fact of popping a needle in doesn't disturb me. I mean I know it's a prick, and it's sort of unpleasant, and if you can't get a needle in the first time, it becomes even more unpleasant because they, you know, get anxious.

Compared to suffering brought about by cancer and the impact of chemotherapy, inflicted pain received little attention from nurses. In the context of hours or days of nausea and vomiting, altered appetite and energy levels, and the anxiety associated with chemotherapy and its effects, venepunctures were seen as momentary and insignificant. While nurses recognized that unsuccessful venepunctures increased patients' anxiety, they saw the associated pain as both minimal and unavoidable. When asked to consider possible ways of alleviating it, nurses either did not see a need to do so or regarded the only means to be injected local anaesthetic, which they felt would inflict more pain than it would relieve.

NURSES' PERCEPTION OF PAIN RELIEF

The work of pain management is complex, with changing needs, difficulties in selecting the most appropriate means of pain relief, and shifting goals. In the absence of objective measures for any of these parameters, relief of pain can easily become subject to individual nurses' judgements, preferences, knowledge, and time constraints. The Burn Care Unit did not have a written protocol or standards for pain management, and the unwritten rules were not necessarily followed. For example, nurses often mentioned that patients should be given Morphine intravenously prior to the first saline bath, the first dressing change after skin grafting, and changes of any particularly large and "difficult" dressings. This perception, however, was not supported by the findings of the study, with two patients receiving no opioids of any kind throughout their time in the Unit, and two further patients receiving no other opioids than a single intramuscular injection at the time of admission to the Unit.

Minimizing the use of strong analgesic drugs

The established routine in the Burn Care Unit was to offer patients milder oral analgesics on 4-hour "drug rounds," which occurred from 7 o'clock in the morning until settling time at around 10 o'clock at night. The drugs of choice were Paracetamol™ or a "cocktail" of Aspirin and Paracetamol™, Panadeine™, or Acupan™. Any additional pain relief, particularly in relation to dressing changes, depended on the individual nurse assigned to care for the patient on a given day. While there were differences between nurses, opioids were generally used sparingly and in relatively small and definitely infrequent doses. Often the determining factor was not the reported intensity of the patient's pain but the timing of the various activities a nurse had planned for her working day. The aim was to make pain *bearable* rather than to reduce it to as minimal a level as possible. The following exemplar illustrates one nurse's decision making in relation to a patient on the day of her admission to the Unit with 15 percent burns some 8 hours after her accident:

> [At around 5 o'clock] she said she was starting to get sore again, and that was about the time when she could have had another injection. About 4 or 5 hours had lapsed [since her last dose of pain-relieving medication]. So we gave her two Panadol™ then, only because we wanted to keep the Morphine until her dressing....Because I wanted to do her dressing at 8 o'clock....If we had given her Morphine at 5, given her another lot of Morphine at 9, and then it would have been too late in the evening....It took us an hour or so [to do the dressing]....Too late in the evening for the dressing.

The patient's experience at this time was of severe, burning pain, yet the medication provided was that suggested as suitable only for mild to moderate headache or musculoskeletal aches (Fields, 1987, p. 272). The Morphine eventually given 3 hours later, prior to the patient's first dressing change, was administered intramuscularly and, at 5mg, amounted to only half of the prescribed dose.

A similar decision (even though for somewhat different reasons), to use a mild oral analgesic instead of an opioid, was made at 8 o'clock the following morning when the patient again reported severe pain. In the following exemplar, an enrolled nurse describes how her more direct and specific knowledge of the patient was overruled by a senior nurse's perceived expertise. The patient's previous dose of analgesic medication, Morphine 10mg, had been given at 4.15 am:

> She said it was getting quite sore again. I had a look at what she'd had. She had some Morphine, and I actually asked [senior nurse] what she felt I should give....She said, "Try her on some Panadol™," which did tide her over, but we have just given her a cocktail [of Aspirin and Paracetamol™]....I would have actually given her Morphine.

> (Why would you have done that?)

> I just felt...my assessment of it...I felt she warranted it.

[Still rather uneasy about going along with the senior nurse's decision despite her own different judgement, the nurse went on to justify her deferential behavior.]

She is far more experienced at it than I am, so I took her word; we would try that. But...I wouldn't leave her in there if I felt that she really did need an injection. Twenty minutes to half an hour later, if she was still in agony I would have done something more about it.

At least two important issues related to nurses' use of pain-relieving drugs arose from the study and are captured in their starkness and simplicity in this exemplar: the first is the ease with which a nurse may be swayed to give the least potent rather than the most potent analgesic drug available to a patient barely 24 hours after her accident and still in severe pain; the second is the more subtle change in the nurse's perception of when administration of Morphine may be justified. Initially, the patient's report of increasing pain and her own assessment of the patient *warranting* opioid medication may have been sufficient. Now it seems that to warrant an injection of Morphine the patient's pain has to be persistent, extreme and obvious. It was such seemingly small incidents that reinforced for both nurses and patients the need to accept pain as inevitable and something to be endured and opioid medication as something to be avoided and used only in dire situations. The not-so-subtle message from the senior nurse was that Morphine should not be used as the first choice, even for severe pain. *Trying* mild oral analgesics in situations of severe background pain, however, not only failed to relieve as much pain as could have been relieved, but it also made it more acceptable to *try* less potent analgesics during episodes of inflicted pain, as in the following example:

I've given her tonight a couple of lots of Acupan™. I don't know if they had given them to her earlier in the day, I haven't actually checked that up. She said that they were quite good during the day. They sort of held her [pain] off. But she was asking me...when she had her Acupan™...if she would be getting an injection because she had an injection yesterday before both dressings. So perhaps they won't be sufficient....I guess I will give her two Acupan™ [before the change of dressings] and see how they go. If not, we can settle her [to sleep, later] with an injection.

Such *trying to see* if a milder drug would work meant that patients often had to endure painful procedures with inadequate analgesia. By the time it became apparent that the medication given was in fact insufficient, it was often considered to be too late to do anything about it. Even when opioids were given, the doses were often too small and insufficient to relieve patients' pain. The following exemplar illustrates the reasoning involved in giving only half of the prescribed dose and then withholding further medication, despite the patient's obvious discomfort and pain. The following situation occurred 4 days after the patient was admitted to the Burn Care Unit with 25 percent burns:

> He really did seem to be in a lot of pain....I knew it was going to take a long time to do....I wanted to give him some Morphine before hand....I thought the Morphine might help relax him before I take down the dressing and put him in the bath....I assumed that 5mg of Morphine [intramuscularly] would have been enough....He was *really* uncomfortable when we had finished the dressing and we had returned him to bed. In fact, he was waiting for the next 2 hours to be over and done with so he could have another injection which would help relax him.

> (Why did you decide that you had to wait this long for the next dose?)

> Well, he can have up to 10mg of Morphine. I could have given him another 5mg after the dressing, but I thought 5mg wasn't effective enough before the dressing, so 5mg won't touch him now. If he could have waited another couple of hours, which seems a long time, which it is, and then I could have given him double the dose, rather than giving him 5mg at one point in time, then 5mg 2 hours later, then another 5mg 2 hours later.

Estimations of drug effectiveness

Nurses in the Burn Care Unit expressed considerable uncertainty as to how effective drugs were in preventing, minimizing and relieving pain. The small, infrequent doses of opioids given to patients would suggest that some nurses overestimated the effectiveness and duration of these drugs. Invariably there was concern about the patient becoming *sleepy* and *doped up* as the result of opioid pain relief, and this was often used to justify the small doses. The following exemplar from the field notes shows the nurse deciding to give less than a third of the prescribed dose of Morphine and, despite indications of pain, retrospectively evaluating her decision as appropriate:

1.30 pm

Patient given 3mg Morphine IV; Nurse stating that 5mg would have been too much. Followed immediately by chest physiotherapy, patient being turned and his (burned) chest being percussed.

1.40 pm

Moved to treatment room for a saline bath and change of dressings.

Patient squeezing his eyes and fists tight as moved from bed to trolley. "Sore!" gasped out between breaths. Lowered into the bath. He held his breath and appeared "winded" as he was lowered into the water. As Nurse started pouring water over his burned back, his whole body became rigid and his face contorted. (The most vivid expression of sheer agony I have ever seen.) Mouth open wide and the whole face contorted in a silent scream. Then cried out "Jesus!" Face went greyish-white in colour (even though he is Maori).

2.00 pm

Given oxygen via a face mask. No explanation. Nurse is using forceps as a scraper to scrape dead skin and scabs off the larger burns on the arms.

Nurse: "How is it going?"

Patient: "OK."

Patient's forehead covered in perspiration. Another nurse supports his right arm while First Nurse scrapes, picks off and debrides dead tissue.

Nurse: "Are you warm enough?"

Patient nods, but does not respond verbally.

2.20 pm

Nurse: "Well, you will be pleased to know that we are almost finished."

Patient: "The worst is still to come."

Nurse: "What's that?"

Patient: "Getting back to bed."

Nurse: "Oh no, we still have to do your dressings."

2.22 pm

Patient raised out of the bath on the metal trolley. Oxygen mask removed. Dried by the two nurses working swiftly. Helped to sit up and large dressings spread with Silver Sulphadiazine™ cream applied to his back. At this point he said he was feeling *faint* and *woozy*. Nurse then asked him to move to a chair [so that she could finish applying the dressing to his back]. He whispered, "I can't," and was left on the trolley. Face ashen and covered in perspiration.

Patient: "I can't take any more."

Nurse: "You have to." [No further conversation]

Dressings to back, arms and foot completed at 2.50 pm, and patient returned to bed.

In the interview immediately after, the nurse stated that she felt that the procedure had *gone well* and the patient had *coped adequately*. She considered that the 3mg of Morphine the patient had been given was sufficient and that he did not need the additional 2mg she had kept on hand, "just in case it was needed. Too much Morphine would have made him too doped up to be able to cooperate." She estimated his pain to have been "not bad, not horrific or anything like that. I asked him if he was OK. If he had said no, I would have given him more [pain medication], but he didn't. I like looking after him. He tries to help himself...he is doing well."

On the other hand, there were nurses who, whether they gave analgesic medication or not, remained skeptical as to whether the drugs made any difference at all. They either believed inflicted pain to be such that no amount of any medication, bar general anaesthesia, would control it or that some patients did not have any *real pain* and could cope without analgesic drugs. Their perception was that patients either did not need or did not benefit from analgesic drugs, even prior to extensive dressing changes. The following exemplars are drawn from a general discussion about pain relief in the Burn Care Unit with two nurses. Their comments relate to a patient with 35 percent burns who was given no pain-relieving medication prior to a 2-hour bath and change of dressings procedure:[2]

> Quite frankly, I didn't even think about it. You see so much pain relief being used here, and honestly, it makes no difference. Patients still cry and scream and say it hurts, so what's the point? Morphine would have made her sleepy but not really helped much.

> When she had the Morphine she was just zonked out. I don't think she has pain. The way she has been burned, it's all deep, it doesn't hurt any more. It's uncomfortable and an effort for her, but I don't think that it's painful for her.

Perhaps because nurses did not expect analgesic medication to make any significant difference in how patients responded to pain, they often assumed that patients had been given all the medication they were prescribed and could safely have. Another assumption was that the provision of pain relief in the Burn Care Unit was more generous than in other areas of the hospital. It was assumed that patients had been given and had taken medication on the regular "drug round" and that, therefore, they could not be given further medication, even when they reported severe pain. As one nurse expressed it,

> I think a lot of people do have pain here; I am talking about general surgery, not burns. I think we do quite well with the burns pain relief.

[but in the same interview]

> Sometimes you are just about afraid to ask them because you know they are going to say, "Oh yes, it's still really painful," and you know you've given them all you can.

Patients who continued to request pain-relieving medication were perceived as *relying on drugs to cope* with pain rather than relying on their own resilience and will to endure. The latter attitude was clearly preferred by the nurses, while reports of pain by patients who were seen as *relying on drugs* (particularly opioids) were treated with some skepticism, or even disregarded. Such patients were considered to be at serious risk of addiction and were even less likely to be given opioid medication. The less experienced nurses who were more likely to give in to patient's requests for pain relief did not necessarily challenge others' assessments. Even patients who clearly needed strong pain relief were seen as *dependent on drugs* rather than in genuine need of relief from real and distressing pain.

In one patient's case, for example, the continuous infusion of Morphine was stopped on his arrival in the Burn Care Unit. Skin grafting surgery to his extensively burned back was postponed for over a week because of his slow recovery from smoke inhalation. Despite daily baths and dressing changes, ongoing severe pain, and his requests for pain relief, he received a total of only 73mg of Morphine in small divided doses over a period of 8 days. This amounted to less than 12 percent of the Morphine he was prescribed and could have received. His own assessment of milder oral analgesic drugs as insufficient during this time was taken as an indication of *not coping* rather than of inadequate pain relief:

> If I had been looking after him the first couple of days he had been in, I would have liked to have given him say Morphine for about the first 4 days, not so much every 4 hours, but every 6 hours at least....I know that he felt that it was the only thing which was working. He was saying that. I gave him an injection [of Morphine] one time because he was in a lot of pain; he was really worked up....He said he hadn't slept for a good 36 to 48 hours, and I could believe that. He was just getting so worked up and couldn't sleep, and sleeping tablets wouldn't work, and no one was listening to him. Everyone was just saying, "Breathe deeply," and he was getting sick and tired of hearing this. I don't think he was really addicted to it [Morphine] because he said to me that I was the only one who had given him an injection over the past few days. And it's not as if he had wanted it for the sake of wanting it....He knew it would relax him and help him go to sleep, at least remove some of the tension that he was feeling at the time.

Even this nurse, however, diagnosed the problem as one of patient anxiety and basic inability to cope rather than as a situation of inadequate pain relief:

> He is coping with pain a lot better now. I think initially, when he came in, he didn't cope very well....I felt that he was very reliant on having the needle because he said that Acupan™ and Panadol™ and nothing else seemed to work.

The whole area of pain relief was fraught with problems and difficulties for the nurses and the patients. Nurses did not feel that the medications they had at their disposal provided the answer to patients' pain. Overall, they considered that drugs, particularly opioids, were dangerous to patients, making them sleepy, unable to cooperate, and at risk of addiction as well as ultimately ineffective in relieving pain. The patient's role in pain relief was ambiguous. When they did not request analgesic medication or give unequivocal evidence of being in pain, their need for pain relief was either inadequately met or overlooked altogether. When, on the other hand, they expressed their needs clearly and specifically, they ran the risk of being misunderstood, once again failing to obtain adequate relief of pain.

Nurses' perceptions of inflicted pain as inevitable and of pain relief measures as less than adequate required that nurses develop ways of dealing with situations of pain infliction in their everyday work.

STRATEGIC RESPONSES TO PAIN INFLICTION

The lived experience of nurses in the Burn Care Unit was that they spent large parts of their working day around people in pain on whom they were required to perform treatment procedures likely to cause further pain. They did not see themselves as having the power to change this situation, either by eliminating the need for the treatments or by eliminating the associated pain. Yet at the same time, these nurses wanted to get some satisfaction from their work; they wanted to feel that they had done something worthwhile for others. To achieve such a sense of satisfaction, nurses had to either succeed extremely well in reducing the amount and intensity of pain they inflicted and maximizing the amount of pain they relieved (*involvement in a therapeutic partnership*), or they had to distance themselves from the patient for a time, making his or her pain invisible (*detachment and objectification*).

Involvement in a therapeutic partnership

One approach to being in a situation of pain infliction was to enter into a *therapeutic partnership* and work closely with the patient. In such a case, the nurse would begin by explaining to the patient what the procedure would involve, listening to patient's fears and concerns, discussing how the patient might participate in retaining significant control in the situation, and usually providing some analgesic medication before commencing the procedure. She would then monitor the patient's responses closely so that additional analgesia could be provided during the procedure. The guiding principle of this approach was that while some pain was unavoidable every effort should be made to keep the pain within the limits the individual patient was willing to tolerate at the time. The nurse-patient partnership depended on the nurse's willingness to become involved in the patient's subjective experience and on her skills in helping the patient share with her the lived experience of being vulnerable and in pain.

In the following exemplar, the nurse makes clear her concern for the patient's subjective experience and her aim of working with the patient so as to share the control over pain infliction and pain relief. The patient was undergoing a saline bath and change of dressings to her hand and leg:

> Initially, when I went in there, I felt that she could cope with what we were actually going to put her through in terms of pain level because I had spent some time with her prior to actually getting her into the shower, and I'd discussed with her what I was going to do, what we were expecting, and the fact that she was going to be in control of the situation. If she felt that it was going to be too uncomfortable, that she could let us know, and that she could take charge. I think that was quite important to her, to feel that she had control....I had actually prepared her to let me know what she needed in terms of her pain relief....It was really a case of assessing it as we went through it, step by step. I think she coped very well with the shower itself. The hand was a bit more stickier than I had anticipated it being, so that was actually a bit more distressing for her than I had hoped it would be....When she made the statement that she was starting to be uncomfortable with it...she was getting a wee bit agitated...a wee bit tense with the whole thing. So at that stage I felt she really did need to have some pain relief. So that's where we were at when she had some [more] pain relief.[3]

> I think it was important to maintain that trust with her. I had already made the statement that she had control of the situation and that she was to let me know when she felt it was more than she could handle. I think I could probably have got away with taking off [the final layer of the dressing], but I think it was important when she had indicated that she couldn't cope any more with what was happening that I, at that stage, went and did something about it....Perhaps another day it would not have been relevant, but today, given the history [of a very painful procedure on the previous day], the time spent and her state of anxiety anyway and the development of a relationship between the two of us, that she could actually trust that what I said was what I was going to do.

[After the Morphine had been given] I felt that we would just take it slowly....She was obviously a lot more comfortable, more relaxed...so it was just a case of listening to her and waiting for indications from her as to how effective the pain relief had been. I wasn't prepared to go in willy nilly and assume that because she'd had that pain relief I could just rip off the paranet [dressing] and we would be set. Because it doesn't always work that way. You don't get total pain relief simply because it's been given intravenously.

In the above account, the nurse shows acute awareness of the close inter-subjectivity between her own and the patient's experience of inflicted pain and its alleviation. Her clinical judgement and actions also demonstrate sensitivity and expertise. This particular exemplar captures best the idea of the *therapeutic partnership* witnessed during the study. In it the nurse accepts the inevitability of some pain, but she carefully works with the patient to ensure that such pain remains within limits acceptable to that person. Just as important, the nurse recognizes the patient's lived situation: that is, her experience from the previous day and the resulting anticipatory anxiety and her need to retain some control in the situation and be respected as a person who matters, who can trust and can be trusted. Rather than seeing the patient's anxiety as a barrier to effective pain management, the nurse recognizes the extent to which it contributes to the experience of pain and the extent to which the growing trust between them can relieve the patient's anxiety. Instead of a subject-object relationship, the nurse is able to foster a therapeutic partnership with the patient and, in the process, reduce the painfulness of the experience for the patient and increase her own sense of satisfaction and accomplishment.

Detachment and objectification

A very different approach to that of therapeutic partnership was also observed. Basically, it involved nurses working on the patient, concentrating on the technical tasks at hand rather than the person. In such situations, pain was also accepted as inevitable, but whereas in a situation of partnership the patient decided what pain was tolerable, here the patient was not consulted. As a consequence, the patient's subjective distress was largely ignored, and there was little evidence of empathy or compassion from nurses during the performance of the pain-inducing tasks. It was not only that some pain was inevitable, but that any pain that the patient experienced was inevitable and did not need to be treated, or could not be treated. The following exemplars are chilling in their acceptance of the inevitability of pain and the degree of detachment nurses were able to achieve in their work with people in pain:

> Well, I knew what I was going to do. And really, there wasn't a lot of feeling behind it. It was a task, and I just set about doing it. I didn't see it as...I know it's pain...you get her in the shower and it's painful, so you try to take her mind off it. You just chat and get it done as quickly as possible....You go on not thinking really. You've got your task and you sort of become like a robot. You go in and chat away and take her mind of it while you are doing whatever you have to do. Get it done.

> With adults we just expect them to put up with it....They are not going to give them Morphine every 4 hours or IV drip (continuous intravenous infusion of opioid medication) for their dressings. It's just not done here....If you've got a soft nurse who thinks it must be sore, then they are a...soft touch, but we expect the patients to put up with it.

> We knew today that he was to have a first dressing, so before that I know that he will require pain relief. It wasn't a large area, and he has not complained of a lot of pain postoperatively, so I didn't anticipate that there will be too much difficulty doing his first dressing. So I thought he only required oral analgesia, so I gave him two Acupan™. I had planned to do him about half an hour after he had the Acupan™, but with one thing and another, I didn't get to do it then. I think probably by the time I had got around to doing his dressing [2 hours later], it was just that half an hour too late. But I felt that the pain wasn't beyond his being able to cope with. The procedure wasn't going to be a terribly long, drawn out one, and the graft actually looked very good. And so I felt that it was all right to proceed. It was not anything I didn't feel he could cope with, and in fact I think he coped very well.

> (Can you remember what you were thinking as you went through doing his dressing?)

> I remember thinking, "Oh my gosh, it's hurting him, but I'll just keep going because I have to do this now. And he will be all right, I am not going to be doing this too much longer."

(How do you think "the patient" coped with the procedure today? How do you think he was affected by it?)

Well, it certainly hurt him. And he will remember that. But I've reassured him that it's not going to be as bad next time. And I think he coped reasonably well. I am certainly not saying that he didn't feel a great deal of pain; I think he did. [Later in the interview the nurse rated the intensity of the patient's pain at 8 on the 10-point scale.] I think he was actually quite shocked about the physical appearance of his foot....I feel that this morning [he] coped very well with pain. He knew that he was going to have pain; in fact, he did have pain, and I rated his pain as being quite high. I don't know what the long-term effects are going to be of that little episode that we had while I was doing his dressing. But I thought he coped very well with that. Okay, he made some noise...but it was nothing that he couldn't be managed out of, and it did abate, and I think he coped well with that. If he was still going on now and rolling around the bed saying, "Oh the pain...I can't stand it"; obviously he wouldn't be coping.

In adopting these strategies of *detachment and objectification*, the nurses became self- rather than patient-focused. They talked of *psyching themselves for what had to be done* or *talking themselves into getting on with the task*, letting their expert bodily skills take over the technical work while they shielded themselves from the person on whom the task was being performed. They tried and often succeeded in distancing themselves from the patient's personal experience and from the painfulness of pain they were helping to generate. Often, it seemed easier to regard the patient as an object on whom skilled work was done than as a person with whom a difficult experience could be shared. In such situations, nurses inflicted pain, but at the same time, they could not acknowledge patient's distress nor provide comfort when it was most needed.

By contrast, the strategy of *involvement in a therapeutic partnership* required that the nurse enter the patient's experience and provide a situation in which the voice of the person in pain could be heard. The patient could thus influence the nurse's body by having her attention, by influencing the pace of the procedure, and by being consulted. The accomplishment of the technical task could become a shared project between the nurse and the patient, each respecting the other's contribution, while at the same time placing equal importance on tending the wounded body and the person in pain. Within this strategy, the nurse's satisfaction came not so much from a competently performed technical task, although that was important, but from having helped the patient come through the experience of wounding and pain with a sense of personal intactness and achievement. In the midst of pain there was caring and renewing of hope, the regaining of a sense of embodied self and of a personal future.

If changes are to be made in clinical practice that will lead to more effective prevention and management of inflicted pain, then it is necessary to understand nurses' involvement in the generation, amelioration and relief of such pain. By drawing on the lived experiences of both patients and nurses, it is possible to arrive at a more complete picture of the phenomenon of inflicted pain and its essential qualities. In the next (and final) chapter the significance of the study findings is examined, and the implications for nursing education, practice, and further research are considered.

ENDNOTES

[1]The distinctive feature of Pethidine (Demerol) is its relatively short duration of action of 2–3 hours (Fields, 1987, p. 254). The nurse's comments need to be considered in the light of the type and timing of this medication.

[2]Although fully conscious, this patient was considered too ill and distressed at this time to consent to participation in the study. She died 3 days later.

[3]The nurse had stopped the procedure at this point and asked that a house surgeon administer some Morphine intravenously. Within 5 minutes patient received 8mg of Morphine, and after another 5 minutes, the procedure was resumed.

Chapter 7
Clinically Inflicted Pain
And Nursing Practice

Inflicted pain is a common yet little acknowledged and poorly understood phenomenon. That assertion was the starting point for this study, and it has been well substantiated by its findings. Clinically inflicted pain is a problematic experience for those who must endure it as well as for those whose actions generate it. Scientific attempts to define and explain it notwithstanding, pain remains a subjective human experience that resists easy objectification and reduction into a readily measurable set of attributes. With that challenge in mind, the aims of the present study were to engage in phenomenological inquiry into the nature of the lived experience of inflicted pain, to make explicit the particular contextualized experiences of those who inflict pain and those who endure it, and to transform that which is individual and private into a written account with the power to deepen our understanding of the phenomenon of inflicted pain.

The choice of phenomenology was deliberate, reflecting a commitment to exploring the nature and meaning of the phenomenon of inflicted pain in the context of lived experience. Furthermore, nursing itself needs a phenomenological sensitivity to the lived experience of patients' and nurses' lifeworlds and a hermeneutic interpretation that more adequately captures the richness and complexity of human life in the midst of trauma, illness and bodily pain (Benner & Wrubel, 1989).

Phenomenological inquiry begins with the personal experience of people able to communicate their embodied experience to the researcher. This first epistemological transformation by the 34 participants in the study of their inchoate, lived experience into an account that I as a researcher could comprehend can best be understood as a gift without which the study would not have been possible. It is these first-order narratives, parts of which are presented here as exemplars of lived experience, that provide the essential grounding for the interpretations and conclusions drawn from the study.

UNDERSTANDING THE NATURE OF INFLICTED PAIN

Irrespective of its source, pain is a subjective, embodied experience. It takes place in a context rich with background meanings and personal concerns. While the importance of contextual variables has been recognized in some research on pain (Choiniere et al., 1989; Fagerhaugh & Strauss, 1977), the present study is different in that it considers the changes within the person, *the embodied self*, as the most intimate context of the experience of pain. The point at issue is not that the person in pain is confined to a hospital bed or a clinic room, required to interact with a variety of health professionals, or even that he or she is aware of being ill; rather, the point is that bodily changes brought about by cancer or burns situate pain into a body that is radically different from the once familiar, taken-for-granted body experienced in everyday life. Changes in the embodied self involve experiences of dis-ease, of *looking different to oneself and the world*, of *feeling different* and *being different*, of *being overwhelmed*, and of the deep-seated need *to be oneself again*. It is in this context that patients encounter inflicted pain, endure it, experience it as having personal meaning, constitute it and are constituted by it. This, then, is the context from which a description of the essential nature of clinically inflicted pain may emerge.

The phenomenon of inflicted pain: The essential themes

To understand inflicted pain as a lived rather than as an observed experience it is necessary to turn to the thing itself—the immediate, prereflective awareness of life (van Manen, 1990) or, in this case, life in pain. The lived experience provides the starting point for the project of phenomenological description, which in turn leads to hermeneutical interpretation and a written account of the essence of the lived experience. For a patient with burns, for example, the observed experience is one of saline baths, debridement of dead tissue, grafting of new skin, and dressing changes; but the lived experience is of the *hurt and painfulness* of inflicted pain, its *wounding* nature, the ongoing need to *hand one's body over to others* to treat and to wound, and the pressures to *restrain the body and the voice* when in pain in order to retain composure and make it easier for others to do their work. It is in returning to this lived experience that one is made aware of the essential nature of inflicted pain and the possibilities for its impact on the people involved.

The hurt and painfulness of inflicted pain

Perhaps the most obvious, and yet the most likely to be overlooked, quality of inflicted pain is its sheer *painfulness*. Such pain is much more than an unpleasant sensation. It hurts, and it has an immediacy of bodily presence that makes it difficult to ignore and, at the same time, in this embodied sense, impossible to share with others. It is this unshareability of the essential painfulness of pain that creates a gulf between those who feel the pain but cannot relieve it and those who, despite a personal contribution to its genesis, cannot feel it yet retain control over the means of its amelioration and relief. For those whose work involves the performance of invasive and painful procedures, the report of inflicted pain invites doubt about its presence and intensity. The prima facie case that invasive procedures hurt, as does the touching and handling of injured tissues, is often rejected. Instead, the patient is required to provide evidence of being in pain, yet even this evidence is not always believed. It is something of a tautology to keep saying that the essence of pain is that it hurts and that it is *painful*. Nevertheless, the doubt thrown on this simple truth by those who need to believe it before they will provide the necessary relief makes it important to restate that which ought to be self-evident.

The lived experience of the person on whom pain is inflicted is not one of doubt but of certainty about the inescapable presence of pain within a wounded, hurting body. The embodied nature of the painfulness of pain is different from the discomforts inherent in restricted movements or the need to maintain a particular posture. In the patients' lived experience, it is also different from the dis-ease of anxiety, the dread of anticipation, or the fear of mutilation, even though all of these may be present at the same time as pain. Thus, while nurses may doubt another's pain, interpreting it as anxiety, fear, or inability to behave like a mature adult, patients on whom pain is inflicted know through their bodies the essential *hurt* and *painfulness* of pain.

The bodily hurt of inflicted pain, which sets it apart from experiences of fear or anxiety, is particularly evident in the language patients use to describe such pain. As well as speaking of *the painfulness* of pain, such language speaks about the essentially *wounding* nature of inflicted pain.

The wounding nature of inflicted pain

While the hurt and painfulness is an essential quality of all pain, one of the things that sets inflicted pain apart from pathological pain resulting from disease is the *wounding* nature of inflicted pain. It is not only that the invasive procedures that puncture, pierce, cut, or tear living tissue are themselves wounding, but more specifically, the pain resulting from such procedures is also wounding. The body already marred by a disease such as cancer or the trauma of burn injuries, and in the latter case already in pain, is further wounded in the course of diagnostic and treatment procedures. For people who have lost a sense of bodily intactness, new attacks on the body bring both pain and feelings of being exposed and vulnerable to further wounding and further pain.

The observed experience may be of a person having blood drawn for laboratory analysis or undergoing a change of dressings. The lived experience is one of *wounding* and *vulnerability* and, almost always, pain. The observed experience involves medical instruments being used to accomplish a necessary task, but the lived experience is of *weapons*—invading, poking and jabbing, "digging around," and "harpooning" the body, with no protection and no escape.

The *wounding* nature of inflicted pain is particularly evident in the strong and unequivocal language used to describe the lived experience. The language is a poignant record of the prereflective, raw experience of pain that "burns," "sears," "stings" and "hurts" in a "horrible," "excruciating," "exhausting," "distressing," and sometimes "overwhelming" way (see Table 4.1). It is also a language of forceful metaphor, trying to make visible the invisible and share the unshareable. People in pain, hoping to have their pain relieved, depend on such language being heard, on being able to communicate clearly and unambiguously the nature of their experience, and on engaging others in the task of relieving the pain. Metaphorical language serves as a means of having the lived experience of *wounding* "lifted into the visible world" (Scarry, 1985, p. 13), a means of making the experience matter to others, especially those able to stop the wounding and relieve the pain.

Whatever its origin, all pain is characterized by hurt and painfulness. This, then, is its first and most pervasive characteristic. The second one is the essentially wounding nature of pain, which stands out in relation to inflicted pain, but is not necessarily limited to it. Nevertheless, it is the wounding quality that sets inflicted pain apart from pathological pain; it is the quality that makes inflicted pain what it is.

Handing one's body over to others

A further integral feature of *clinically* inflicted pain in adults is the patient's consent to and involvement in the generation of such pain. The pain of physical assault, torture, or self-harm have the qualities of painfulness and wounding, but they do not typically require the person to willingly *hand over his or her body to others* to hurt and to wound. In the clinical context, however, this is an essential component that makes possible the infliction of pain and sets limits on how the person in pain can act in the situation.

The essence of clinically inflicted pain is not only that *the pain hurts me* or that *the actions of another hurt me*, but that *I invite the pain by making my body available to another to wound and to hurt*. As discussed earlier, handing one's body over to others is not a passive process of acquiescence; rather, it requires that patients allow others free access to their bodies, knowing that such access is likely to result in pain, while at the same time keeping sufficient control over their bodies to retain outward composure and not hinder others' work. The lived body, with its intentionality, can facilitate others' work, or it can act as an obstacle, frustrating such work and making pain more likely. Thus, while it is the actions of another that inflict the pain, the patient is not a passive bystander to the event of pain generation. It is not only that he or she must endure the pain, but in presenting a marred, damaged, uncooperative, or in some other way inadequate body, the person becomes implicated in the generation of pain.

The body that has lost its integrity through burn injuries is more *woundable* and open to the possibility of pain. The mere exposure of such a body to air, water, or ordinary touch creates the potential for pain. Similarly, the patient with cancer who presents an arm swollen with lymphoedema or veins made fragile by past exposures to chemotherapy is made aware of an inadequate body that must bear some of the responsibility for the pain inflicted on it. Hence, clinically inflicted pain involves not only another's actions on *my* body, but also *my* inability to present an adequate body that would not impede the work of another.

Restraining the body and the voice

Part of handing one's body over to others involves retaining adequate control over the body so that it does not impede the work of others. Our habitual being in the world tends toward avoidance of pain, and yet, in the clinical situation, this inclination must be overcome and the body restrained so that it remains available to those who must work on it. Furthermore, clinically inflicted pain not only results from actions of others, but much of it must be endured in their presence. As a result, the social situation in which clinically inflicted pain must be endured creates its own imperatives, including the requirement that the patient behave with composure and cooperation. To do otherwise would not only interfere with the work of others, but would challenge the legitimacy of their actions as well as the patients' willingness and ability to keep to their side of the implied contract. The patients' work is to endure and to do so in a way that facilitates rather than hampers the work of others.

By *restraining the body and the voice,* people in pain exercise a degree of control over themselves and their world. Situated in an unfamiliar, hostile world in which disease and injuries, contingencies of treatment, and the will of others dominate, they need to hold on to that which is still under their control. Thus, *restraining one's body and voice* is a means of asserting control over a shrinking sphere of personal influence, in this case one's body (however affected by disease and injuries) and one's communication with the world (however unresponsive that world might be to the person's needs and desires).

According to Scarry (1985, p. 19), intense bodily pain is "language-destroying," deconstructing complex prose into a series of preverbal moans, whimpers, and screams. It is a frightening prospect, for to be reduced to this level of being and communication is to lose the dignity and sense of worth inherent in being human; it is to be dehumanized. *Restraining the body and the voice* is, thus, an essential aspect of enduring clinically inflicted pain and its legitimized wounding and destructiveness. But the experience is more complex than that. When present, the voice has the power to influence the shared situation, to force others to take notice; when absent, it allows those who inflict pain to define the situation in their own terms, by-passing the lived experience of the person in pain. Thus, *restraining the body and the voice* is an essential way of being in pain that facilitates the work of others and allows the person to maintain outward composure while at the same time adding to the ultimate unshareability of the experience of pain.

A comment on the four essential themes

Of the four essential themes that describe the nature of clinically inflicted pain (its *hurt and painfulness,* its *wounding nature, handing one's body over to others,* and *restraining the body and the voice*), some are shared with other types of pain, while others are specific to this condition. The *hurt and painfulness* is the essential quality of all pain, regardless of its genesis or circumstances. The quality of *wounding* may be present in different types of pain, but it is especially evident in the case of any inflicted pain, whether in the context of clinical treatment, assault, war, or torture. These two aspects of clinically inflicted pain are inherent in pain being pain and in the wounding nature of another's actions that create the pain. In other words, the pain has an existence of its own: that is, it is within the body of the person, and yet, it is independent of the person's intentions.

What gives clinically inflicted pain its particular quality is the nature of involvement required of the person on whom pain is inflicted. It is the voluntary nature of the *handing of one's body over to others* to wound and to hurt and the voluntary (even though also socially expected) efforts to *restrain the body and the voice* from offering resistance or complaint that distinguish clinically inflicted pain from other forms of inflicted pain. The nature of personal involvement in the clinical situation both invites the pain and cedes control over its duration and intensity to others. Thus, *handing one's body over to others* and *restraining the body and the voice* are not incidental to the pain or merely aspects of the patient role; rather, they define the nature of the lived experience of clinically inflicted pain in which personal consent and cooperation must be present.

When personal consent and cooperation are withheld, that is, when the person resists making his or her body available to others and makes no effort to restrain the body and the voice, then the very nature of the situation is changed. This difference makes more comprehensible the distinction that nurses in the study drew between working with adults and working with children and the stress they experienced when inflicting pain on children. Unlike adults, children do not usually voluntarily *hand their bodies over* to be hurt and wounded, and neither do they necessarily *restrain their bodies and their voices* (Offsay, 1989). As a result, their bodies are restrained against their will, and as far as possible, their voices are ignored or the meaning reinterpreted as indicative not of pain but of fear and the inability to grasp the good intent inherent in the actions of others. The coercive nature of the situation means that *terror* as well as pain is inflicted and the line between therapy and assault is blurred. In such situations, nurses may reason that their actions are necessary, therapeutic, and therefore justified, but the patients' behavior provides forceful evidence of the harm being done to the person. To be permitted at all, restraining the patient's body against the person's will and persisting with a procedure despite his or her protestations have to be constructed as therapeutic in intent and outcome. The immediate experience, however, is of wounding and pain forced on a person who is not free to refuse them. Such a situation may give rise to the ethical question of the patient's right to refuse treatment when the pain caused against the patient's expressed wishes may be seen as violence rather than therapy.

Thus, clinically inflicted pain is defined not only by the objective legitimacy of the therapeutic situation, but even more so by the personal involvement of the patient on whom pain is inflicted. It is the nature of the social situation in which it occurs, which requires both a therapeutic intent from the person inflicting the pain and active cooperation from the patient, that makes inflicted pain distinctive.

UNDERSTANDING THE EXPERIENCE OF INFLICTING AND RELIEVING PAIN

The phenomenon of clinically inflicted pain presented here emerged out of the patients' experiences. For them, inflicted pain was first and foremost a direct, embodied, elemental experience, grasped as meaningful in terms of its immediate hurt and painfulness. It was also an experience that they tried to understand and interpret in its broader context as deserved or undeserved punishment or, more frequently, as simply an unavoidable part of their present situation.

The nurses who inflicted the pain, on the other hand, did not and could not have direct experience of the patients' pain. They were aware of the patients' expressions of pain and, when they attended to such expressions, of their own sense of dis-ease and stress in the situation. Even then, their familiarity with how patients behave when having venepunctures or undergoing burn dressing changes often made what they witnessed ordinary and "normal." From their perspective, the pain was perceived as expected, inevitable, and largely intractable.

Tactile encounter and pain infliction

The exigencies of treatment bring the nurse and the patient into close physical contact with each other, and it is in the context of a tactile encounter between them that pain comes into being. The tactile encounter also demonstrates their separateness and their very different views of the experience of pain. The nurse is the one who touches; the patient the one who is touched. But the touch which they share often lacks a quality of empathic intent that would bring them together in a shared understanding of what each is experiencing; rather, the touch is instrumental, determined by technical purposes, often breaking through the boundaries of the patient's physical body, penetrating and invading and bringing pain into the patient's bodily space. As this study has demonstrated, there is a risk that the nurse will objectify the person on whom pain is inflicted and that the nurse-patient encounter will be reduced to a technical performance that brings about pain for the patient but little mutual understanding.

Even though the risk of objectification and detachment became the reality in many instances, this study also demonstrated that the tactile encounter, the arbiter of pain, could be organized in a very different way. The instrumental, technical purposes still dictated *what* needed to be done but not *how* it was to be done. Patients in particular appreciated nurses who, in their encounters with them, demonstrated *gentleness* and *sensitivity*, *trustworthiness* and *technical expertise*, and the ability to inform, reassure, and make the person feel special. Nurses in this study demonstrated these qualities in the midst of what patients experienced as painful procedures. That nurses could achieve this quality of caring and involvement, despite also having to inflict pain at the same time, speaks about the complex nature of nursing practice and points out the ability of nurses to attend to both the technical task and to the person. It is in the context of inflicting and relieving pain that we can see both evidence for and the difficulties in the view of nursing as "a caring practice whose science is guided by the moral art and ethics of care and responsibility" (Benner & Wrubel, 1989, p. xi).

Caring and inflicting pain

Wanting to care and having to inflict pain are dissonant and not easily reconcilable facets of nurses' work with patients in acute hospital settings. In the absence of collective responses and help, individual nurses are left to resolve the dissonance for themselves. Sometimes, as in the case of oncology clinic nurses, this may mean deciding to leave the situation by moving to another clinical area. For other nurses, the dissonance may lead to personal feelings of weakness and inadequacy and attempts to emulate more experienced colleagues in their apparent clarity of purpose and ability to focus on the technical requirements of the task at hand.

For a nurse new to the experience of inflicting pain, the dissonance comes from two sources. First, in order to accomplish the task that she knows to be painful to the patient, the nurse distances herself from the person on whom the task is performed. Such distancing and detachment help her to accomplish the task, but they also leave her dissatisfied, knowing that she had, however temporarily, failed to be present to the patient in a caring and supporting way. "Being mindfully present" has been identified as an essential component of nurses' expression of caring (Euswas, 1991), and yet having to inflict pain makes such a quality of being-with the patient more difficult to achieve. Second, and perhaps more important, there is an inner conflict between the nurse's emotional desire to respond with compassion to a fellow human being and the rational argument that convinces her of the necessity to inflict pain. This inner dichotomy is difficult to sustain, and there is the risk that the compassionate response will be suppressed, robbing nursing intervention of its human warmth and feeling and thereby dehumanizing both the patient and the nurse.

However justifiable the pain we must inflict, we should never forget that all pain hurts. When inflicted with technical detachment and without feeling or regret, pain dehumanizes not only the person who must endure it, but also the person who inflicts it. In the end, the dangers are perhaps greater for the one who inflicts the pain than for the person who endures it. In arguing against moral rationalism, which ignores the contribution of embodied human emotions such as sympathy and compassion as motives for moral action, Prior (1989) warns that

> reason cannot "argue us out of" our compassion for human suffering; it can, however, harden us to that suffering by preventing us from acting as our emotions dictate....In time, this pattern of "rational" action could lead to the suppression not only of compassion but [also] of the guilt that results from that suppression. (p. 37)

This is not to suggest that compassion is devoid of a rational component or that one must choose between reason and emotion in determining moral action; rather, it argues for the need to recognize the significance of both reason and compassion working together in safeguarding the humanity of those who suffer pain and those whose work requires that they inflict it.

There are real dangers in clinical situations in which technological needs supersede nurses' desire to practice "caring as a moral art" or where "avoidant strategies interfere with compassionate care, and can cause an emotional numbing that can reach all aspects of the nurse's life" (Benner & Wrubel, 1989, pp. xi, 377). Nurses may come to see detachment as a necessary and justifiable prerequisite to their own survival in the situation of pain infliction. Reflecting on the conflicting demands of wanting to care and having to inflict pain, Tisdale (1986, p. 126) observes that

> without this detachment, the pain strikes you in the face like a haymaker, like an unexpected splash of cold water. That visceral urge to be rid of it—to *make it go away*—would win out. To stay on the job you have to be able to hold up the trembling leg, hold down the struggling child, and think of other things.

Yet the situations in which the only choice nurses feel able to make is to *become like a robot, block out* [patients' responses], *get quite hard to it, put on a steel face,* and *not blink an eyelid...detach [one]self from the person for a time, while it hurts* create a breach not only between the nurse and the patient, but also between the nurse as a person and her being-in-the-world. To inflict pain on a daily basis and train oneself to feel nothing of the other's pain is to be diminished as a person; it is to compromise one's own sense of wholeness and moral responsibility and one's commitment to the centrality of caring in nursing practice. Such concerns have far-reaching implications for the quality of patient care and for the nurses themselves, and they are too important to be left to individual nurses to struggle with in the privacy of their consciences.

Involvement in a therapeutic partnership

The phenomenological approach used in this study has uncovered the risks and problems inherent in nursing practice that distances itself from the essential nature of inflicted pain. It has also made alternative choices and possibilities clearer. Such alternatives demonstrate recognition of the lived, embodied reality of pain; they point out the need for nurses to imaginatively and compassionately enter the patients' reality, to become sensitive to each patient's concerns and situated possibilities, and to create opportunities for collaborative action in the joint project of reducing pain and suffering.

The paradigm case of *involvement in a therapeutic partnership* captures the essential qualities of nursing practice guided by a view of nursing as caring action. It demonstrates that caring involvement is needed, and possible, in the midst of pain infliction, and it illustrates the centrality of involvement rather than detachment in inflicting pain and the need to keep it within the patient's self-determined levels of tolerance. It is also an example of an "expert nurse" (Benner, 1984a), empowering a frightened and dependent patient and helping him/her to regain confidence in his/her shattered world.

In the case of a therapeutic partnership, the nurse demonstrates *concern* by recognizing the patient's need for information, for involvement in his/her own care, and for control over how much pain he/she is able to endure and with what assistance. The nurse uses both *generalized and specific knowledge* to inform the patient of what will happen during a lengthy and quite likely painful procedure, what the patient may expect, and how the patient can be involved in the situation. The *uniqueness of the person* is recognized through the acknowledgment of his/her need to be in control and to determine if and when he/she may need further analgesia.

What is obvious in this situation is that the nurse is concerned not only with accomplishing the task or with gaining the patient's cooperation, but from the beginning his/her actions demonstrate concern for the person and the quality of the experience that he/she will share with the patient. The nurse uses his/her power in the situation not to reduce the patient to an *object* on whom work is to be done, but to empower the patient to become actively involved as *body-subject*, whose voice and body can communicate the lived experience otherwise hidden from the nurse. The nurse not only invites the patient to share his/her (patient's) lived experience as it unfolds, and so is able to become involved in it, he/she trusts the patient's account and acts on it. It is the nurse's trust in the patient's account of pain that lays the foundation for the patient's trust in the nurse as a person who can be relied on not to go beyond what the patient feels able to tolerate at a particular time.

Throughout the painful procedure, the nurse remains attentive to the patient's evolving experience, attuned to the verbal and bodily signs of increasing pain. He/she does not try to convince the patient, or him/herself, of the legitimacy and inevitability of the pain being inflicted; rather, the nurse focuses on helping the patient live through the experience by alleviating pain, reducing feelings of vulnerability, and building up the trust that the patient will need in order to be able to face future episodes of painful treatment. The nurse does not demand or expect stoicism and courage from the patient. He/she accepts anxiety as the patient's way of being in the situation, made more understandable by the history of pain already suffered, and the nurse adapts his/her actions to change the situation and thus increase the patient's confidence in it. The nurse's involvement is based on sound scientific knowledge (of pain and the effects of analgesic medication) and compassionate concern for the person. There is no suggestion of the nurse becoming "overinvolved" or immobilized by the patient's experience; rather, the nurse offers the kind of solicitude that facilitates and empowers the patient "to be what he or she wants to be" (Benner & Wrubel, 1989, p. 49). This, in essence, is what phenomenologically informed nursing practice is and can be.

The problem of undermedication for pain

The frequent undermedication for pain observed in the Burn Care Unit is one further area of the study findings that requires particular mention. Like pain, undermedication for its relief is not always easy to define or to assess objectively. Individual patients require different amounts of analgesic medication to provide what they would subjectively regard as adequate relief. In a general sense, undermedication may be said to occur when patients are left to endure significant pain while not being provided with pain-relieving medication at a level established as effective and safe through research and systematic clinical observation. In practice, this often means that the patient is prescribed suboptimal doses of analgesic medication or is given such medication in doses that are smaller and less frequent than those ordered by the physician, despite reports of significant pain.

The study produced extensive evidence of less than optimum medication for pain. Given previous research in the area (Bonica, 1980; Choiniere et al., 1989; Perry, Heidrich, & Ramos, 1981), this finding was not unexpected. What was unexpected was that neither patients nor nurses in the present study perceived their situation as one of undertreatment or undermedication for pain.

Despite the often severe pain they experienced, patients in the Burn Care Unit did not perceive their situation in terms of undertreatment. The idea of undertreatment or undermedication requires general knowledge of what is possible, specific knowledge of what is being done, and an appreciation of the disparity between the two. Patients in the study did not have and were not given the information they would have needed to make a judgement on this matter. As noted earlier, the small numbers of patients with burns in the Unit at any one time meant that they seldom had access to other patients with similar injuries with whom to compare progress and evaluate their own responses in the situation. Unable to make comparisons with others, patients could learn only from their own embodied experiences and from nurses. In this context, their embodied awareness was of pain and of the need for relief. At the same time, they did not have technical knowledge concerning analgesic drugs or optimum strategies that could have been used to relieve their pain. Even when they did acquire embodied, experiential knowledge, such as the awareness of the greater effectiveness of parenteral Morphine when compared to milder oral medication, patients were not usually able to use such knowledge to obtain more effective pain relief. Despite this, patients maintained an attitude of benevolence toward nurses, "a predisposition on the part of patients to think well of the nursing staff" (Christensen, 1988, p. 325). They viewed nurses as the experts who would use their knowledge to do their best for patients. Thus, they gratefully accepted what medication was provided, but they seldom questioned nurses' decisions about the choice and dosage of drugs or decisions to withhold analgesic drugs altogether. Instead, they accepted the need to endure whatever pain was left as a necessary price of being healed, a stance reinforced by nurses and their views on inflicted pain.

What was particularly striking about the nurses' perceptions of the pain-relieving measures used in the Burn Care Unit was their acceptance that things had to be as they were and that they as nurses had to learn to live with the status quo. The prevailing values of minimal use of analgesic drugs, particularly narcotics, were not challenged openly and therefore did not change, even when individual nurses acted against them on isolated occasions. Adherence to the status quo prevented nurses from considering alternative and more effective approaches to pain prevention and relief, such as the use of inhalation analgesia, continuous intravenous infusions of Morphine or Fentanyl™, or patient-controlled analgesia by means of intravenous pumps (Bryan-Brown, 1986; Fitzgerald, 1989). In turn, lack of exposure to alternative means of pain relief helped to reinforce the present situation. Thus, while patients continued to report severe pain, nurses generally considered that adequate pain relief was being provided or that nothing further could be done to alleviate the pain. Their belief that they were doing all that could be done to relieve patients' pain made it both easier for them to feel a sense of job satisfaction and more difficult to perceive a need to change the status quo.

The use of a phenomenological approach in this study has facilitated some understanding of the way peoples' situations and background knowledge shape the way in which they construct their experiences. Thus, it is possible for both patients and nurses to be engaged in a situation in which severe pain is experienced and insufficient medication provided and yet never raise the question of undermedication.

LIMITATIONS OF THE STUDY

Limitations may be seen as restrictions or shortcomings and, thus, as negative attributes that diminish the object to which they are applied. The term may also be used to denote more precisely the scope of something, its legitimate boundaries, and the extent of its application. Some important limitations, largely in the latter sense of the word, are recognized in the design, methods used, and presentation of this study. Their acknowledgement at this point should assist the reader to appreciate more clearly the scope of this study and to take a more informed stance in assessing the implications of its findings.

This investigation adopted a clinical orientation rather than relying on poetry, drama, painting, or other sources of potential data for a phenomenological study of inflicted pain. This decision may have limited the scope of the book that has been developed as the result of the particular research undertaken, but by its clear clinical focus, it has also strengthened the outcome and made it more applicable to nursing practice.

Another limitation relates to what may be perceived as the desired, or ideal, standards in phenomenological research and what it is possible to achieve given the constraints of the researcher's own lifeworld. By its nature, phenomenological inquiry requires conditions that can facilitate ongoing dialogue between the researcher and the participants in the study, not only during the period of initial data collection and analysis, but also during the much longer period of reflection, interpretation and writing. Phenomenological research also tends toward open-endedness. In other words, it often starts with a broad question, which is only refined in the process of research, and needs to draw its data from a broad range of sources. Furthermore, the research process needs to be flexible since the boundaries, whether in terms of numbers of participants, sources of data, or time needed to complete various phases of inquiry, cannot be specified accurately in advance. Ideally then, the researcher should be free to respond to the developments of the research as and when these occur.

However, since time and resource constraints inevitably arise, pragmatic decisions must be made. In the case of the present study, some of the open-endedness in the research process had to be sacrificed in order to meet the time and resource constraints imposed by the terms and conditions for completion of a PhD. For example, although they were at different stages of illness experience, none of the patients with cancer who took part in the study had cancer-related pain. Thus, their experience of pain was limited almost exclusively to venepunctures and other investigative procedures. It would have been helpful to know whether given more experience with pain from other sources their perceptions of clinically inflicted pain would have been different. However, due largely to time constraints, it was not possible to extend the study to either continue data collection with these patients or to recruit additional participants. Therefore, individual readers must judge the "fittingness" of the findings (Sandelowski, 1986) to situations outside of those that were described in this study.

An additional limitation of the study is the extent to which the findings were able to be validated with the participating patients and nurses. While such validation is often advocated in phenomenological research (Campbell, 1986; Riemen, 1986a), it is not always practicable or possible. The difficulties of contacting individual participants after a span of more than 2 years needed to write up the findings were anticipated. Therefore, particular care was taken to validate early interpretations with individual participants in final interviews with them. I also provided feedback and conducted two group interviews with nurses at the conclusion of my time in the field. Later, during the process of writing, findings were shared and discussed with a number of nursing colleagues, including those with clinical and research expertise. Their critical and validating comments were taken into account in the writing of the final draft of the thesis that was developed into this book. While the lack of validation of the study's findings by the people on whose experience the research is based is recognized as a limitation (Miles & Huberman, 1984; Sandelowski, 1986), it is not one that could be easily overcome.

A further (though less clear) limitation relates to the conditions under which data analysis and interpretation were undertaken. Literature on qualitative research points to potential disadvantages of data analysis and interpretation *a cappella* (i.e., working alone) (Stern, 1991, p. 147) as opposed to within a research team or using expert "judge panels" (Brink, 1991, p. 172). Stern, however, also notes potential difficulties with the use of expert panels since not having participated in the data collection they often lack contextual sensitivity, and not having been fully immersed in the data, they often lack full knowledge of the data and data categories. Within the present study, the thesis supervisors were always available and helpful in their feedback, providing opportunities for what van Manen (1990, p. 100) has termed "collaborative discussions," questioning, pointing to weaknesses, and helping to bring out strengths. Ultimately, however, the work of analysis and interpretation was done *a cappella*. In part, this reflects the reality of PhD study within New Zealand universities (and their British traditions) where the candidate works independently rather than as a member of a research team. It also illustrates the relative dearth of experts in phenomenological research (particularly within nursing) in New Zealand and the difficulties faced by a researcher wishing to pursue innovative and pioneering work. In order to overcome these difficulties, aspects of the thesis were presented to students and colleagues for discussion and comment as well as at two international and two New Zealand conferences. Also, two internationally recognized nurse-researchers provided critical comments on the first draft of the thesis. While any qualitative study done *a cappella* may be open to the criticism of idiosyncratic interpretation, in this case (and in addition to other measures already outlined), every attempt has been made to document "a clear decision trail" and facilitate "auditability" of the research report (Sandelowski, 1986).

Furthermore, if one accepts van Manen's (1990) contention that in phenomenology "writing is our method" (p. 124) and the very essence of doing research, then expert panels may have an important, but limited, contribution to make to the ultimate quality of hermeneutical interpretation. Others may advise and critique, but it is the writer who authors the text and makes public understandings and insights achieved through a long and sometimes lonely process of turning to the phenomenon, investigating the lived experience, reflecting on it, interpreting it, and bringing it to speech.

IMPLICATIONS OF THE STUDY

In a preface to her commentary on Merleau-Ponty's *Phenomenology of perception*, Langer (1989) states that

the existentialist philosophers' central concern is to prompt humans not to live thoughtlessly but rather, to have a keen awareness of their freedom and responsibility in the shaping of a situation in which they are always already involved. (p. ix)

In a more circumscribed fashion, and with a focus on nursing practice in the context of pain infliction, my concern within the present study is to challenge nurses to practice more thoughtfully: to be sensitive to the patients' and their own lived experiences, to recognize the power they have in inflicting and relieving pain, and to exercise the freedom and responsibility they have in a way that enhances comfort and demonstrates care.

The world of nursing and the world of pain often intermingle. As this study has shown, nurses have the power to relieve pain and suffering, but they are also required to perform tasks and procedures that generate pain and add to patients' distress. To say that an action *generates pain* sounds simple and unproblematic, so we add comments about "suffering" and "distress" to ensure that the point is not lost, that it conveys its intended message. The temptation is to doubt the reality of pain and its essential painfulness, to see it as limited to "a few seconds or minutes" or to "only the prick of a needle" or "only the edges of the graft" or to see it as inevitable. All of these perceptions cocoon the nurse into a world apart from the patient's lived experience. Yet, as this study has shown, the possibilities for pain amelioration and relief do exist, as do the different possibilities for being-with and acting-on the person in pain.

Implications for nursing education

A major question that arises out of the present study is the extent to which nurses are educationally prepared for practice that requires them to knowingly and regularly inflict pain on patients in their care. Just as important is the question of how much and what kind of help nurses already in clinical practice receive in learning to respond to situations of pain infliction. The response needs to include care of the patient as well as personal coping, which each nurse must engage in if he/she is to retain a sense of personal and professional integrity. Thus, the study raises implications for nursing practice as well as for both basic and continuing nursing education.

The nurses who participated in the study did not feel that their nursing education had prepared them to cope with the lived reality of having to inflict pain in the course of their work. There is no reason to believe that their experience is unique, yet, if nurses are to be prepared for the reality of practice that awaits them in many settings, particularly acute care settings, then the issue of clinically inflicted pain needs to be examined in the educational preparation of nurses. If they are to be helped to become skilled and caring practitioners, then students of nursing need to learn that their intentions of engendering feelings of comfort, safety, confidence and hope, and relief from anxiety, fear, and worry may not always be realized. There will be times when they will be required to carry out treatments or provide interventions that carry a potential to wound, cause discomfort and pain, engender feelings of vulnerability, and increase fear and anxiety. If patients' experiences are not to become a matter of chance or oversight, then the nurses need to be able to intervene in a way that recognizes the risks and the potentials in a situation. More specifically, nursing curricula need to address the problem of inflicted pain, the barriers to management and relief of such pain, the impact on nurses of inflicting pain in the course of their work, and the dangers of becoming insensitive to patients' suffering.

Educational programs need to assist students by facing the ethical implications of inflicting pain "for the patient's own good" and by addressing questions such as "How much pain should a patient be expected to endure?" and "Who should decide what the limits of tolerance ought to be in any given situation?" Consideration of these issues will not resolve all the questions nor obviate the need for nurses to learn from their own and others' experiences in practice. Nevertheless, it might present a more complete and realistic picture of nursing practice and, just as important, demonstrate acceptance of the problem of clinically inflicted pain as a collective concern rather than a personal difficulty that individual nurses must resolve for themselves.

Students need to learn that in situations of clinically inflicted pain nurses travel a narrow road between compassion and detachment (Tisdale, 1986). They must acknowledge the pain they themselves generate and will go on generating while at the same time retaining a caring and compassionate relationship with the people they are hurting. Finding a balance in such situations is not easy and requires maturity and a complex range of knowledge and skills.

Nurses need knowledge of the mechanisms of pain, the relationships between tissue damage and inflammatory processes and the ensuing nociception and pain, as well as, the relationships between wound healing, scar formation and pain. They also need knowledge of analgesia and, in this context, particular knowledge of pharmacological means of pain relief. More specifically, nurses need a clear understanding of the pharmacokinetics of the drugs they use as well as their particular strengths, limitations and associated risks. Sound knowledge based on research rather than folklore is needed to dispel "opiophobia" (Morgan, 1986), unfounded fears of addiction, and other myths that surround the use of narcotics in the context of acute pain (Angarola, 1986).

The absence of any nonpharmacological techniques for pain relief in the present study suggests a need for education in the use of complementary analgesic strategies. A wide range of psychological and cognitive-behavioral therapies might be useful adjuncts to pharmacological analgesia. Nurses need to develop skills in using such therapies and in deciding what combinations of pharmacological and other strategies might be appropriate in specific situations. Relaxation and guided imagery as well as the use of music have been shown to be useful adjuncts to pharmacological analgesia in many situations of clinically inflicted pain (Angus & Faux, 1989; Blotcky, 1986; Jay et al., 1986; Tobiasen & Hiebert, 1985). Hypnosis has been shown to be effective in reducing different kinds of pain, including pain related to burn debridement (Orne & Dinges, 1989; Wakeman & Kaplan, 1978). While these measures are not uniformly successful, nurses do need to be able to use all the tools at their disposal to provide optimum care both in preventing and in relieving pain, no less so when the pain results from their own actions.

By increasing the range of possible responses to a situation, technical knowledge is essential for nursing practice in the area of pain management. Yet on its own, technical knowledge is clearly insufficient. Nurses also need the ability to examine ethical issues that arise out of their practice. Nursing education programs need to facilitate the development of ethical reasoning in their students and provide them with the opportunities to consider ethical questions related specifically to the infliction of pain and its relief.

Nurses in the present study often justified inflicted pain as an *inevitable consequence of necessary therapeutic procedures*. They did not intend to cause pain; rather, pain was the consequence of a "good" action performed to a "good" end. Thus, the traditional doctrine of the "principle of double effect" (MacKinnon, 1988, p. 324) may be said to apply. In other words, if the intent is to do good (cure a person from cancer), then an unintended evil side effect (pain) is permissible, providing that the good consequences (cure) outweigh the bad ones (pain). Even when this principle is accepted, questions remain.

For example, can all clinically inflicted pain be justified on this basis? How is the "good" of one consequence to be measured against the "evil" of another, and who should do the measuring? However intellectually challenging they might be, such questions need to be seen in their practical application since in practice, and with varying degrees of reflective awareness, nurses answer them through their actions. As a result, patient's autonomy may be enhanced through what the present study has described as a *therapeutic partnership* and what Gadow (1986) refers to as an "advocacy partnership" (p. 21), or it may be lost amid paternalistic assumptions that the professionals "know best."

The ethic of partnership requires the fostering of collaborative rather than competitive or hierarchical nurse-patient relationships. It also requires the *sharing* of decision-making, planning of care, and evaluation of progress. Above all, it requires that control over pain, its infliction, duration, management, and relief be *shared* between the nurse and the patient. The nurse can then "coach" and support the patient through frightening, painful, and distressing experiences (Benner, 1984a, p. 89), lending his/her wisdom and strength, and empowering the person in pain to retain a sense of control and personal integrity in a situation that might otherwise lead to helplessness and despair. Such therapeutic partnerships must be built on mutual trust and a willingness to expose personal vulnerability and weaknesses since the line between what a patient feels able to endure and what a nurse knows she cannot relieve is narrow and seldom clearly defined.

However, as the study has also shown, when autonomy and self-determination are suppressed for the "good of the patient," paternalism may take over, and patients can be exposed to more pain and less pain relief than, given adequate information, they would choose for themselves. Nurses who lack the knowledge to act in a more effective fashion, who accept the status quo as the only possibility in the situation, and who feel forced to choose between sensitivity to patient's needs and self-preservation can easily fall victim to the ethic of paternalism. Rather than sharing control with the person in pain, the nurse (unwittingly perhaps) submits to paternalism of others and reinforces its powers by acting without consultation with the patient, simply assuming the benefits of his/her actions.

There would also be value in educational programs that address ethical issues related to the prevention and relief of inflicted pain. For example, how vigorously should nurses try to prevent and relieve pain? In the present study, nurses favored the minimal use of pain-relieving measures and emphasized stoical suffering and endurance. More specifically, patients were often encouraged to "cope" with severe pain without "relying" on analgesic medication. While some patients may choose stoical endurance for themselves, a question that needs to be asked is whether nurses have a right, or perceive themselves as having an obligation, to try to instill the stoic values of courage and silent endurance in patients who lack them or choose not to demonstrate them (Edwards, 1984). Without adequate consideration of such ethical issues, nurses may fail to develop the depth of understanding necessary to create situations of therapeutic partnership evident in the practice of those nurses in the study who recognized the patients' pain and worked closely with them to alleviate it. Instead, like other nurse participants, they may remain focused on their own feelings and their own needs for protection from "infectious identification" with the patient (Gadow, 1980, p. 91), thereby distancing themselves from the patient's pain and adopting an attitude of detachment.

Given the dichotomy that often arises between the patient's lived experience of pain and the scientifically constructed nature of nurses' knowledge about pain, there is also a need for nurses to learn something about the intersubjectivity of human experience. In other words, nurses need to learn how to attend to another's experience of pain, without becoming either overwhelmed and immobilized by it or detached and immune to calls for help. Nurses need to not only listen to their patients, but to learn from them since only patients can teach them about their (patients') lived bodies, things that matter to them, and the ministrations that they find appropriate and helpful. The ability to combine technical knowledge and clinical expertise with attentiveness to the lived experience of the patient allows the nurse to develop understandings that are attuned to patients' subjective experience.

A number of nursing writers have stressed the centrality of *lived body* and *lived experience* to nursing practice and nursing curricula (Benner & Wrubel, 1989; Gadow, 1980; Lawler, 1997). What they also emphasize is the need for nurses to expand their horizons so that they can learn how to relate their scientific knowledge to the lived experience (of pain) in a way that recognizes both the uniqueness of the lived experience and its intersubjectivity within shared understandings (of what it is to be ill, to suffer and to be in pain). Much of this material cannot be learned in the classroom or from extant nursing theory; instead, it must come from context-specific experiences, from experts who are able to coach novice nurses through the work that needs to be done, and through the responses they will experience in the process of their work. The experts are patients who know personally what it is to cope with inflicted pain and nurses who acknowledge fully that they inflict pain and yet practice nursing in a caring, thoughtful way.

Didactic teaching of broad principles is only a beginning. Nurses need to learn not only the techniques of sterile dressings or venepunctures, but also how to perform these procedures in such a way that they cause the least possible pain. When invited to share their experience, patients can teach new nurses how to perform a procedure such as skin debridement while causing minimal pain or how to decrease the pain of an unsuccessful venepuncture. Through role modeling, an expert nurse can teach another nurse how to develop a therapeutic partnership with a patient, sharing control over pain infliction and pain relief, building trust, relieving anxiety, and respecting the patient's right to determine his/her own level of pain tolerance. Such context-specific, first-hand knowledge is discovered in practice, but it needs to be shared with others in order to demonstrate the complexity of nursing work and the possibilities for excellence in caring and the ongoing learning present in every nursing situation.

Implications for nursing practice

To have pain inflicted in the course of medically prescribed treatment is to feel hurt, wounded, vulnerable and afraid while at the same time having to hand one's body over to others to work on and restrain the body and the voice from their habitual being. This situation, perhaps more than any other in nursing, calls for a thoughtful, reflective practice that recognizes fully its freedom and its responsibility.

The first and the greatest need is for nurses in practice to recognize the nature and extent of their involvement in the infliction of pain. Because nurses experience pain infliction as a difficult and stressful aspect of their work, there is always the temptation to rationalize or redefine it as necessary, as inevitable, as perhaps not hurting as much or as long as other kinds of pain, or as nonharmful and even beneficial to patients' recovery. Such redefinitions mask the essential nature of inflicted pain, that is, the patient's lived experience of its painfulness and its wounding and the effort required to submit to it and to endure it. They are attempts to make pain less real by rendering it invisible and manipulable by the language in which it is described. Yet, as Merleau-Ponty (1962) states categorically, "The world is not what I think, but what I live through" (pp. xvi-xvii). In other words, the redefinitions have the potential to reduce the reality of the other's pain to what *I think* is possible, but they are not necessarily true to the essential nature of pain. Pain is first and foremost an embodied experience. Unless there is open acknowledgment by nurses of the lived nature of inflicted pain, then their practice will fall short of its full potential. Reconstructing patients' pain, without doing enough to alleviate it, may make the situation more tolerable for nurses, but it will not ease and indeed may increase patients' experience of pain and suffering.

Nurses in clinical practice need greater knowledge of pain and its impact on people who must endure it. In particular, nurses in clinical practice need to recognize the difference between *nociception* and *pain*. Tissue damage caused by procedures such as venepunctures, the removal of dressings that pull away damaged or newly granulating tissue, or the scrubbing of the raw wound or exposing it to heat or cold are all practices that have the capacity to produce the noxious stimulation of the sensory nerve endings and, thus, nociception. Nociception involves activation of peripheral nerve endings by chemical, mechanical, or thermal energy and transmission of information to the central nervous system by means of electrochemical nerve impulses (Fields, 1987). Pain, on the other hand, is a subjective perceptual experience that results from activity in the central nervous system, which can be affected by anxiety and other emotional states, altered by analgesic and other types of medication, or eliminated by the use of local or general anaesthesia. Thus, while nociception may be an inevitable consequence of many nursing procedures that involve some degree of tissue damage, pain is not, unless nothing is done to prevent nociception from becoming pain.

Nurses also need more specific knowledge of the patients with whom they are working so that they can develop a quality of understanding of the patient's situation, personal meanings, and coping strategies. They also need to develop knowledge of patients' bodies, not only in their objective sense (e.g., having "lymphoedema" or "6 percent full-thickness burns"), but as lived bodies, exposed and vulnerable under the gaze and touch of others.

One way in which such specific knowledge may develop is through greater continuity of care, for example, through primary nursing. When there is a lack of continuity of care, as in the Burn Care Unit in the present study, then patients are often exposed to nurses who do not know the extent of their injuries, the healing that has taken place, the areas that may be particularly sensitive and painful, or the signs that would indicate how well individual patients are able to tolerate the pain being inflicted. Without such specific knowledge, there is the risk of "simply getting on with the job," focusing on technical performance, and overlooking the lived experience of the patient. At the same time, there is a need to recognize the stress inherent in having to inflict pain and the need for nurses to be able to step back from a situation that taxes their capacities to act with sensitivity and care. Primary nursing should not be used to leave individual nurses to cope in isolation with the demands of seriously ill patients and the lengthy, painful procedures that must be performed on them. Instead, the greater continuity of care afforded by primary nursing should be used to provide more sensitive and more individualized care while providing assistance and support to primary nurses during the particularly stressful periods of exacting work.

The findings of the present study indicate that patients experienced considerable and, at times, extreme pain, yet the amount of analgesic medication they were given was often minimal and inadequate to relieve the pain. A great deal of the nurses' efforts were directed not so much at the relief of pain as to the encouragement of patients to control the expression of their pain and to endure it without "reliance" on drugs. These findings are not exceptional; rather, they confirm what many other researchers have found in similar contexts (Choiniere et al., 1989; Fagerhaugh & Strauss, 1977; Perry, 1984c). Therefore, a crucial step toward better management of inflicted pain must be improved knowledge of analgesic medication and its use in specific areas of clinical practice.

Nurses' attitudes toward the use of pain-relieving medication also need to be questioned. For example, authoritative advice on the care of patients with burns is that opioids are the mainstay of pain management, not only during the initial few days, but for as long as tissue damage (i.e., nociception) remains (Marvin & Heimbach, 1985). These authors advise that adult patients should be given Morphine *intravenously* in doses of *10–15mg* and that such dosages should be continued for procedural pain until wound healing is complete. Research studies have indicated that average doses of 6.5mg (Choiniere et al., 1989) or even 8.9mg of Morphine (Perry et al., 1981), administered prior to treatment procedure for burns, did not provide adequate pain control. Despite such evidence, patients in the Burn Care Unit in the present study were often given no more than 3–5mg of Morphine intravenously or 5–10mg intramuscularly or none at all for fear of too much sedation or risks of addiction. The fear that opioids would make patients sleepy or "zonked out" needs to be challenged and examined.

Tisdale (1986) suggests that when nurses deprive patients in pain of opioid pain relief they are "protecting them from the possibility of pleasure, of dreamy rest, of absence and release" (p. 193). In fact, patients in the present study who were given Morphine did not report pleasure, or even freedom from pain. At best, they experienced some dulling of pain during the procedure and the temporary relief of "nonpain" once they were left to rest in the safety of their beds. We need to ask whether protecting patients from the risks of addiction, known to be minimal in "normal" persons (Fields, 1987, p. 264), justifies the inadequate relief of ongoing and often severe pain. Once again, there is a need to recognize the "primacy of caring" in nursing practice and the need for clinical decisions and actions to be "guided by the moral art and ethics of care and responsibility" (Benner & Wrubel, 1989, p. xi). Nurses need to recognize that however vulnerable they may feel patients undergoing painful procedures entrust their very bodies to them, handing them over to be wounded and hurt. Nursing response to such trust needs to be one of thoughtful care and responsibility, not only for the quality of their own technical performance, but for the quality of the patients' lived experience.

There is also a need in all nursing settings for periodic reviews of current practices and accepted protocols related to pain management. Case reviews might highlight inconsistencies in pain assessment, prescribing, and management as well as the effects of individual nurses' preferences for particular forms of pain relief. Such reviews might also provide opportunities to examine the ethical values and reasoning operating in the situation, something that did not occur in either of the two settings used for the study. In particular, there is a need for nurses in practice to be aware of the growing body of research literature on the topic of pain management, to be informed about the recent improvements in pharmacological and other means of pain relief, and to be prepared to evaluate their own practice and its outcomes. Clinical leadership, whether from charge nurses, clinical nurse specialists, or expert senior nurses, must be present if nurses in practice are to provide the best possible care for people in pain.

Implications for further research

The previously noted dearth of qualitative research in the area of clinically inflicted pain and its management suggests that the first and most significant implication of the present study is the need that it has shown for such research. Phenomenological research begins with the lived experience and brings to reflective awareness those aspects of the lifeworld that scholars, researchers, and even those living the experience often overlook or take for granted (van Manen, 1990). This bringing of the phenomenon of clinically inflicted pain to reflective awareness raises a number of issues for future research. The issues relate to pain, to other subjective experiences commonly encountered in acute care settings, to broader aspects of nursing work, and to the selection of research methods in studies of experiences of illness and nursing practice.

The present study leaves unanswered some specific questions related to clinically inflicted pain that deserve further research: for example, What is the lived experience of clinically inflicted pain like in other clinical settings such as emergency rooms, intensive care units, surgical wards, or maternity units? How do nurses in those settings perceive inflicted pain and their role in its generation, prevention and relief? Additional questions arise when broader implications of having to endure inflicted pain are considered: for example, What are the long-term effects of having to hand one's body over to be wounded and hurt? How can patients be helped to retain or recover a sense of personal embodiment altered through repeated experiences of clinically inflicted pain? How are children's lived experiences of such pain different from those of adults, and what are the ramifications for nursing practice?

The question of cultural values and norms in relation to pain infliction and pain endurance deserves particular attention: for example, How culturally embedded is the need to restrain the body and the voice in situations of clinically inflicted pain? This is just one question that arises out of the present study. Other questions might address the issues of cultural understandings and crosscultural communication as well as the possibilities that inflicted pain may be enhanced by institutional practices based on prejudice and racism rather than sensitive recognition of cultural differences in pain tolerance and pain expression.

Furthermore, encouraging nurses to become involved in therapeutic partnerships with patients on whom they must perform painful procedures or warning them of the undesirability of distancing and detachment is not enough. We need better understanding of the *background knowledge, situated meanings* and *personal concerns* (Benner & Wrubel, 1989) that motivate and enable nurses to develop high levels of rapport with their patients and assist them to practice in qualitatively different ways. In particular, there is a need for research into expert nursing practice in the context of pain, including clinically inflicted pain.

The explication of the phenomenon of clinically inflicted pain raises questions about the need for similar phenomenological studies of other types of acute and chronic pathological pain from the perspective of lived human experience: for example, What is it like to suffer the pain of migraine, endometriosis, chronic arthritis, or different kinds of trauma? Related to this is the question of how well nurses working with people who endure such pain know and understand their patients' lived experience and what practices they employ to relieve such pain.

Furthermore, the present study provides a possible model for phenomenological research into other lived experiences that are an important part of human life in situations of health and illness. Such phenomena may have received little attention in nursing research to date, but they are (or should be) of immense practical concern to nurses: for example, What is it like for busy working women to live through weeks of "morning sickness" in early pregnancy in the context of personal and social values that stress that pregnancy is a "normal" biological event? What is the lived experience of ongoing fatigue like for patients with chronic renal or respiratory disease, those receiving chemotherapy for cancer, or the terminally ill? What is the impact of chronic fatigue on the patient's perceptions of embodied self, on family relationships, and on other aspects of the person's being-in-the-world?

If there are important aspects of patients' lived experience that require further research, careful explication, and deeper understanding, there are also important aspects of nurses' experience that deserve similar attention. Benner and Wrubel (1989) state that

> nurses provide care for people in the midst of health, pain, loss, fear, disfigurement, death, grieving, challenge, growth, birth, and transition on an intimate front-line basis. Expert nurses call this *the privileged place of nursing*. (p. xi)

As the present study has shown, however, the demands on the nurse who occupies such a privileged place can be considerable. Nurses may be emotionally and morally burdened by their patients' experiences, by others' decisions, and by their own actions when they have to engage in practices that contributes to patients' discomfort, pain, and suffering. *Involvement in a therapeutic partnership* is one possible option in such a context. *Distancing and detachment* is another option. No doubt there are other choices. Further research is needed to explore nurses' embodied experiences of their practice worlds, of the ethically and emotionally complex situations in which caring is mediated by hurt, wounding and pain, and of the nurses' experiences of learning and developing expert practice in such situations. Phenomenological research may be particularly effective in capturing the complex nature of such context-specific experiences that need to be understood in order for others, particularly less experienced nurses, to learn from them.

Nursing practice is much more than a collection of particular actions or processes. It is an ongoing activity of being-with those who are ill, hurting, vulnerable, afraid, or in some other way in need of nursing care. Some research questions that arise out of nursing practice might be of the problem-solving kind. In such cases, experimental studies may be needed to determine the relative benefits of a particular technique or intervention. Very often, however, as in the case of the question that started this study, the issues are different, requiring a different research approach. With its focus on the lived experience, its openness to the unexpected, its aims of understanding in context, and its promise of insights into that which we often take for granted, phenomenological research has much to offer nursing research and nursing scholarship. Because it always "begins in the lifeworld" (van Manen, 1990, p. 7), phenomenological research may be particularly responsive to clinical issues and situations that call for a contextual understanding and reflective, thoughtful practice.

CONCLUSION

The work of Merleau-Ponty has been central to this study, and the thesis which has developed from it. The phenomenological imperative of *returning to things themselves* was crucial in focusing the inquiry away from "the abstract and derivative sign-language" of traditional science (Merleau-Ponty, 1962, p. ix), evident in most of the earlier research on pain, and to the lived experience of those who know pain in an embodied, personal way. Turning to lived experience has made possible the description of the essential qualities of the phenomenon of clinically inflicted pain in a language that is both analytical, and yet, close to that used by the study participants. It has also made possible the use of exemplars, which ground the analysis and interpretation in the lifeworld of elemental human experience and capture the essence of what it is to endure inflicted pain or be involved in its generation.

The study has also utilized the central phenomenological idea of *the lifeworld* as the context of lived experience. Lifeworld is much more than the world of physical objects, people and events. For Merleau-Ponty (1962), lifeworld is that through which we live and through which we come to know ourselves. For the patients in the study, the key features of their lifeworld were the tactile encounters with nurses and other hospital staff, and the impact of lived space and time on themselves, their experiences of pain, and their perceptions of possibilities for coping and for the future. It was in the interaction with the lifeworld, or rather, through their inhabiting that world, that people in pain gained new awareness of themselves and of the meaning the experience had for them. In Marcel's (1984a) words, "The situations help to reveal me to myself." The authenticity of this argument was borne out in the participants' awareness of their changed situation and its impact on their embodied selves and in their ability to describe that experience to the researcher. It was through extended dialogue with the study participants about their experiences that the understanding of clinically inflicted pain as an embodied experience developed. The key themes of *hurt and painfulness, expectation and experience of wounding, handing one's body over to others,* and *restraining the body and the voice* carry the meaning of the phenomenon of clinically inflicted pain. They could not have emerged without due attentiveness to the lifeworld within which such pain is experienced.

It was Merleau-Ponty's exposition of *embodiment*, however, more than any other phenomenological theme, that has informed the understanding and interpretation of the lived experience of clinically inflicted pain in this study. Pain, according to Merleau-Ponty (1962), has a spatiality that places it within the fabric of the body and makes it inseparable from the essential self. If we accept this view, then human pain cannot be reduced to an objective, easily measurable phenomenon, which carries the same meaning regardless of context. Rather, as I have argued in this book, the depth of understanding will emerge only when the context is taken into account.

The four essential qualities of clinically inflicted pain all situate pain within the body. It is in and through the body that people experience clinically inflicted pain and are involved in its generation and in its endurance. The *hurt and painfulness* of clinically inflicted pain is more than nociceptive activity within the anatomical body. Rather, it challenges the familiar, taken-for-granted body of everyday life, entering it, and creating a "pain-infested space" within it (Merleau-Ponty, 1962, p. 93). Further impact on the lived body occurs through *the expectation and experience of wounding*, making the person feel vulnerable and exposed. The essential requirements of *handing one's body over to others* and *restraining the body and the voice*, make it necessary to resist the natural being-in-the-world of the "inborn complex" and the "habitual body," adopting instead a stance of tension and vigilance.

Effective nursing practice in the context of clinically inflicted pain must involve not only technical intervention, but attentiveness to the lived experience of the person in pain and a particular quality of being-in-the-situation. It is by turning to the essentially embodied nature of the lived experience, and the particular lifeworld of the person in pain, that the potential for effective and sensitive nursing action may be realized.

Appropriate and effective nursing interventions depend on adequate understanding of human experiences of health and illness and the meanings such experiences have for the people involved. As this study has demonstrated in relation to clinically inflicted pain, phenomenological research can do much to deepen our understanding of lived human experience and nursing involvement in it. Rather than depending on concepts and definitions from outside, phenomenology encourages and facilitates the study and articulation of human experience and nursing practice from within. Furthermore, phenomenological inquiry reveals nursing as essentially "a human venture with a moral purpose" (Bishop & Scudder, 1990) or, in the words of Benner and Wrubel (1989), as "a caring practice whose science is guided by the moral art and ethics of care and responsibility" (p. xi). What the present study has demonstrated in relation to nursing practice is the significance of *the therapeutic partnership* in situations of pain infliction, built on the ethics of care and responsibility. Thus, both nursing practice and nursing scholarship have much to gain from phenomenological inquiry. In addition, the phenomenological imperative of returning to the lived world of human experience may assist in bringing the two aspects of the discipline of nursing closer together.

Appendix A
The Design, Methods, and Context of the Study

ASSUMPTIONS OF PHENOMENOLOGICAL RESEARCH

The key assumption of phenomenological research is that knowledge of phenomena can be derived from the adequately apprehended experience of those who live the experience (Munhall & Oiler, 1986). In other words,

> The whole universe of science is built upon the world as directly experienced, and if we want to subject science itself to rigorous scrutiny and arrive at a precise assessment of its meaning and scope, we must begin by reawakening the basic experience of the world of which science is the second-order expression. (Merleau-Ponty, 1962, p. vii)

The present study was predicated on the above assumption as a starting point toward a deeper understanding of clinically inflicted pain as a lived human experience. Yet at the same time, there are occasions when phenomenological research may fail in its quest to understand human experience, especially when potential participants are unable or unwilling to adequately communicate their experience to others. To a significant extent, phenomenological research depends on participants' narratives and descriptions of subjective experiences and personal meanings that cannot be accessed directly by the researcher. Therefore, at the outset of the present study, I, as the researcher, was faced with the question of how well patients and nurses directly involved in the experience of inflicted pain could and would communicate embodied experiences.

In choosing the phenomenological path, I had also to accept the second important assumption of phenomenological research, that is, in most instances, people are able to communicate their inchoate experience and practical knowledge of the situation in an honest and trustworthy manner. A significant part of my "turning to the phenomenon" (van Manen, 1984, 1990) involved accepting the phenomenological principle that the researcher needs to approach each participant as someone who, because he or she has direct experience of the phenomenon the researcher is trying to understand, is "an expert on the topic of inquiry" (Swanson-Kauffman & Schonwald, 1988, p. 102).

In entering the field, I had to trust both the research approach, to the extent that it has shown itself to be an appropriate and fruitful method when used by others, and also myself as a person whose presence, sensitivity, and involvement in the situation would affect the quality of the eventual outcome of the study. Phenomenological research depends on "the researcher's ability to engage with the informants' reality" and requires empathy, intuition, and a high level of attentiveness (Swanson-Kauffman & Schonwald, 1988, p. 101). Participant observation and in-depth or "phenomenal interviews" (Massarik, 1981) provide possibilities for an empathic engagement and quality of rapport that are necessary for true understanding. Moreover, the ongoing dialogue between the researcher and the participants, and their mutual involvement in the validation process, highlights engagement rather than traditional scientific objectivity and contextual meaningfulness rather than generalizability (Sandelowski, 1986). In its design and execution, the present study demonstrates acceptance of and adherence to these key assumptions and principles of the phenomenological method.

AIMS OF PHENOMENOLOGICAL RESEARCH

The aims of phenomenology are to understand lived experience and what it means to be human, to delve into the very nature of the phenomena, and to understand human experiences in their contexts and complexity (van Manen, 1984, 1990). Such aims cannot be achieved through the means of the traditional scientific method, guided as it is by existing theory, predetermined hypotheses, and the reduction of phenomena under study to variables and operational definitions. Phenomenology, according to Merleau-Ponty (1962), is not only a particular philosophy and study of phenomena in the world, it is also a particular style of thinking that takes in the complexity of situated meanings and remains true to the lived experience.

Like other research methods, phenomenology aims to transform personal lived experience into consensually validated social knowledge (Lynch-Sauer, 1985; Reinharz, 1983). However, unlike methods of inquiry that neglect to make their particular transformation processes explicit, phenomenology requires that the steps by which direct experience is transformed into a written account and made available to others should be specified. To reach its aim of transforming private experience into public knowledge, phenomenological research requires active involvement not only from the researcher, but also from the study participants and the audience who eventually read and evaluate the research report.

The nature and sequence of epistemological transformations involved in the process of phenomenological research, and followed in the present study, are outlined most clearly by Reinharz (1983):

- The first transformation is performed by the participating person who in the context of a research situation transforms private experience into actions and language and makes these available to the researcher. Such self-revelation requires an atmosphere of trust and mutual respect;

- the second transformation is performed by the researcher who, unable to enter and sense directly another's experience, has to produce his or her own understanding of that experience from information communicated by the participating person;

- having grasped the participant's experience, the researcher then needs to transform it into conceptual categories that capture the nature and meaning of the experience rather than merely recording it;

- the researcher then has to transform the understanding and conceptual categories into a coherent, meaningful account—such as a research report or a conference paper—that makes the knowledge public and open to scrutiny; and

- the final transformation has to be performed by those who have not participated in the research process but who as the audience need to create their own understanding of the phenomenon, clarifying existing understandings and asking new questions about human experience. (pp. 77–79)

Thus, phenomenological research is a creative process, and in each transformation, "something can be lost and something can be gained." (Reinharz, 1983, p. 79). It is an interpretive, inductive process, requiring sensitivity and intuitive skills (Donaldson, 1987), and it should be added that it carries the risk of idiosyncratic interpretation. However, by making the steps of the epistemological transformation explicit, and by describing the context of the experiences under study, the number of possible interpretations is limited (Benner, 1984b; Leonard, 1989), and the reader is better able to determine the validity of the conclusions drawn by the researcher.

The actual carrying out of phenomenological research involves a series of interrelated activities, which, according to van Manen (1984, 1990), include: turning to a phenomenon of concern and interest to the researcher; investigating the experience as it is lived; reflecting on the essential themes that emerge from the investigation; and describing the phenomenon and bringing it to speech.

TURNING TO THE PHENOMENON OF INFLICTED PAIN IN CLINICAL PRACTICE

In line with the general aims of phenomenology, this study focuses on the discovery and understanding of the experience of pain through its systematic examination in the context in which the experience is lived. The field study design was used to allow for participant observation by the researcher in situations where inflicted pain was expected to occur and for interviews with patients and nurses directly involved in such situations. The study was designed to describe and examine patients' and nurses' experiences as they are lived and not to test hypotheses based on existing theories.

Preparation for the study began 12 months prior to the commencement of data collection with the investigation of the selected setting, and it included a period of familiarization with the setting, the staff, and treatment protocols. The 3 days spent in the clinical setting provided the necessary reassurance that the study was feasible and that the staff were willing to facilitate the research. As the result of this period in the field, some design changes were made to the study. For example, oncology outpatients rather than inpatients were included as the majority of patients on chemotherapy are treated on an outpatient basis.

Entering the field

The decision to work with cancer patients receiving intravenous chemotherapy and patients recovering from burns was made on the basis of clinical experience, a literature review, and consultation with thesis supervisors. This decision, in turn, influenced the selection of the particular setting for the study, which was undertaken in a medium-sized, acute care hospital located in a major New Zealand city. The key factor in the selection of the setting was the need for the population from which study participants would be drawn to have direct experience of the phenomenon under study and be able to speak about the experience and express feelings in a language comprehensible to the researcher (Omery, 1983).

Entry into the field was negotiated through the Research Ethics Committee of the Hospital Board concerned and in consultation with the chief nursing and medical administrators of the hospital. The first week in the field was spent largely in formal and informal meetings with nursing and medical staff explaining the study, its purpose and methods.

Assumptions and expectations

My past experience in clinical nursing research in the area of pain (Madjar, 1981), and familiarity with the relevant literature have all contributed to personal assumptions and expectations present at the beginning of the study. I have worked as a nurse in a variety of acute hospital settings, including critical care units, although not in specialized burn care units or oncology wards. Nevertheless, I have personal experience of nursing work and of having to perform procedures knowing that they would probably hurt the patient. On the other hand, my personal experience of inflicted pain is very limited since I have not had surgery or been a patient in a hospital. The most intense inflicted pain I have experienced is that related to dental fillings and extractions.

The phenomenological approach requires that these assumptions and expectations be made explicit and, to the extent that it is individually possible, "bracketed" or set aside (Oiler, 1986; Ray, 1985; Swanson-Kauffman & Schonwald, 1988). In other words, the researcher should reveal conscious personal biases and allow the reader to assess the extent to which these have been recognized and set aside during the study, thus allowing the participants' responses and data to determine the significant issues, questions, and themes of the study. It is always possible that the researcher's expectations will be confirmed, but one should not set out to either confirm or disprove particular expectations or hypotheses. In the case of the present study, the following assumptions and expectations were recognized and, as far as possible, bracketed:

- that patients with cancer receiving intravenous chemotherapy and patients with burns severe enough to require hospitalization will experience some clinically inflicted pain, that such pain may reach high levels of intensity in some circumstances, and that some patients may have difficulties coping with the pain;

- that the need to prevent, minimize and relieve clinically inflicted pain may not always be adequately recognized by nurses and others involved in patient care and that the reasons for this are not well understood. As a nurse, I have been concerned with the issue of inflicted pain and have spoken out about the need for improvements in this area of nursing practice (Madjar, 1987);

- that staff may perceive the study as an unwelcome evaluation of their work and practice and may feel threatened by the topic and methods of the study. It may have been possible to make the study less threatening by presenting it as a broad-focussed study, but my decision was that such a presentation would be both dishonest and impractical; and

- that I should be honest and open about the study, its aims and methods with all participants and that there should be no attempt to conceal the study's focus on inflicted pain.

From my perspective, this last point was particularly important, not only because of the personally held values about honesty in research, but also because of the demands of the phenomenological approach used for the study. When participants are considered active partners in the research enterprise rather than as passive subjects whose only role is to yield information needed by the researcher, then they have a right to be treated as responsible human beings, able to decide for themselves what information they are able and willing to share. Whatever sharing occurs needs to be within an ongoing dialogue based on mutual respect and trust (Farnsworth, 1985). Furthermore, any attempt to validate the findings with the participants, an accepted part of the phenomenological method (Omery 1983), cannot be based on a deception about the true nature and purpose of the study.

Selection of participants for the study

In order to obtain "a purposeful [or theoretical] sample" for the study (Morse, 1989b, p. 119), only those individuals who had direct knowledge of the phenomenon of inflicted pain were included in the study. Rather than in any way trying to obtain a representative sample, in terms of age, gender, ethnic background, or socioeconomic status, patients and nurses were invited to take part in the study on the basis of their experience and ability to share their knowledge of that experience in a research context. Children were not included in the study since they might be different from adults in the way they perceive medical interventions, how they reason about them, and how they express their experiences in language and actions.[1]

Potential patient-participants were approached and asked about participation in the study as they presented at the Oncology Clinic or following admission to the Burn Care Unit on the basis of the following criteria:

- that they were over 16 years of age and able to communicate in English without difficulty;

- that they were admitted to the hospital for treatment of burns requiring changes of dressings, cleaning, debridement, grafting, and/or application of medication to burned areas of the body, or they were attending the Oncology Clinic for diagnostic tests and intravenous administration of chemotherapy, fluids, or blood transfusions as part of therapy for cancer;

- that they had no recent history of psychiatric illness; and

- that they indicated willingness to participate in the study by giving a written consent following the explanation of the study and their participation in it.

The eventual sample consisted of seven patients (two women and five men) with burn injuries and seven patients (four women and three men) undergoing chemotherapy for treatment of cancer. In addition, 20 nurses also participated in the study, 15 from the Burn Care Unit, four from the Oncology Clinic, and one who worked in the diagnostic laboratory and obtained blood samples from both groups of patients.

All 20 nurses were women. Seventeen were registered general or comprehensive nurses, and three, all in the Burn Care Unit, were enrolled nurses (see Appendix B). Because of their more limited education, enrolled nurses are legally required to work under the supervision of a registered nurse (or a physician), but in the Burn Care Unit, they usually carried similar workloads and responsibilities as registered nurses. The main difference was that only registered nurses could take responsibility for administering intravenous fluids and drugs and were also required to check oral medication administered by enrolled nurses. Otherwise, enrolled nurses were expected to formulate nursing care plans, perform dressing-change and other technical procedures, and make judgements about patients' needs for information, emotional support, pain relief and other nursing interventions. (Unless a nursing qualification is significant in a particular situation, no distinction is made between enrolled and registered nurses in the report of the study.)

Some of the nurses had completed specialist inservice courses (in the care of burn and plastic surgery patients), but none of them had higher professional qualifications such as an advanced diploma or a university degree. Nurses were invited to participate in the study on the basis of the following criteria:

- that they had been or were about to be directly involved in the performance of diagnostic or treatment procedures on one or more of the patients included in the study and where the nature of the procedure was such that it had or was likely to result in some pain for the patient; and

- that they indicated willingness to participate in the study by giving a written consent following the explanation of the study and their participation in it.

All of the patients and nurses who met the above criteria and were approached agreed to take part in the study. In the Oncology Clinic, the seven patients who consented to participate were either at the beginning of a chemotherapy treatment cycle or were expected to undergo at least three further weekly or monthly administrations of intravenous chemotherapy. For this reason, two patients who consented to participation but had their treatment altered to exclude intravenous administration of medication following the initial interview were excluded from the study. Patients on oral chemotherapy regimens who did not receive intravenous drugs and whose blood tests tended to be performed less frequently and who therefore experienced less inflicted pain were not included in the study. The focus in data collection was on current experiences rather than recollections of past events. Therefore, a purposeful sampling approach was used to include those patients most able to contribute to the aims of the study (Morse, 1989b; Omery, 1983).

All seven patients with burns who met the inclusion criteria consented to participation in the study. During the time of data collection in the field, a number of children were admitted to the Burn Care Unit as well as six other adults. Of the six adults, one was a recent immigrant who did not speak English, one elderly patient suffered from longstanding confusion and memory loss, one had severe psychotic disturbance, one suffered extensive trauma and died without recovering, and two patients who suffered relatively minor burns were admitted overnight for social rather than specific treatment reasons. While these patients were not included in the study, indirectly they still contributed important background information in that during interviews nurses used examples from their experience, which included past as well as current patients, or made comparisons as a way of clarifying a point being made. The 15 Burn Care Unit nurses included in the study comprised about one half of the nursing staff of the unit and were all directly involved in the care of the patients already included in the study.

All participants were given code numbers, and these codes, rather than names, were used on any material that required transcription by a typist or was discussed with thesis supervisors.

Description of participants

(See also Tables A.1 and A.2 for this information in summary form.)

Burn Care Unit patients

Patient 1 was a 27-year-old male who suffered first-degree burns to his left foot and first and second-degree burns to his right hand and arm (approximately 5 percent of the body surface area) as a result of spilling burning oil at home. He was admitted directly to the Burn Care Unit after first aid, but no analgesic medication was provided in the emergency department of the same hospital.

Patient 2 was a 31-year-old male who suffered full-thickness burns to his right foot and first-degree burns to his right arm (approximately 5 percent of the body surface area) as the result of spilling burning oil and putting out a fire in the kitchen of his home. Initially treated at another hospital and sent home, he was admitted to the Burn Care Unit 3 days later when his foot had become infected and painful.

Patient 3 was a 21-year-old unemployed male laborer. He suffered superficial to full-thickness burns over 25 percent of his body, including face, shoulders, back (from the shoulders to the buttocks), left arm, hands and left foot as well as smoke inhalation damage to lungs and a corneal ulcer on the left eye. He was rescued unconscious from a house fire, required artificial ventilation, and was treated in the intensive care unit of another hospital before being transferred to the Burn Care Unit 4 days later. By this time he was fully conscious, able to breathe spontaneously, and was receiving opioid analgesia via continuous intravenous infusion.

Patient 4 was a 25-year-old male sports facility attendant. He suffered first and second-degree burns to 12 percent of the body surface, including face, head, neck, and arms, from ignited fumes after a friend had poured kerosene on a barbecue. His eyelids were damaged, and he was unable to see for the first 3 days. He was admitted to the Burn Care Unit after receiving first aid, but no analgesic medication, in a community medical centre some distance from the hospital.

Patient 5 was a 53-year-old female education consultant who suffered approximately 6 percent, mainly second and third-degree burns, to her left arm, shoulder and chest as a result of spilling burning wax at her home. She was admitted to the Burn Care Unit after receiving first aid, but no analgesic medication, in the emergency department of the same hospital.

Patient 6 was a 36-year-old female civil servant. She suffered a mix of superficial to full-thickness hot water burns over 15 percent of her body surface, with deep burns to her left hand, right leg and foot and the left side of her face and head. Swelling of the eyelids prevented her from being able to see for the first 2 days. She had suffered from epilepsy since adolescence and was burned as a result of a grand mal epileptic seizure while under the shower at home. She was rescued by neighbors and transported by ambulance to the emergency department of another hospital, where she received first aid, intravenous fluids and opioid analgesia before being transferred to the Burn Care Unit some 2 hours later.

Patient 7 was a 42-year-old male truck driver who suffered burns to 25 percent of his body surface when the petrol tanker he was driving overturned and exploded. His injuries included full-thickness burns to both hands, second-degree burns to both legs and superficial burns to face and neck as well as a broken finger and chest contusion. He also suffered some burn trauma to the inside of his mouth and hot fumes inhalation damage to his lungs. The impairment in his lung function necessitated continuous administration of oxygen via a face mask for 10 days, but he was able to breathe without mechanical ventilatory assistance. He received first aid, intravenous fluids and opioid analgesia at another hospital before being transferred to the Burn Care Unit some 4 hours later.

Oncology Clinic patients

Patient 1 was a 46-year-old female office worker who was diagnosed as having carcinoma of the breast a week earlier. By the time she sought medical attention, a year after first noticing a lump, her left breast was ulcerated and the disease had spread into the lymph glands and the chest wall affecting her right breast and causing severe swelling of the left arm. The breast ulcer was surgically debrided, and she commenced on a course of chemotherapy, including intravenous Adriamycin™ and Vincristine™ and oral Tamoxifen™ and Prednisone™ (see Appendix B).

Patient 2 was a 39-year-old housewife. She was initially treated for lymphocytic lymphoma 2 years earlier, but with the recent recurrence of the nodes in her neck and abdomen, she was commenced on another cycle of chemotherapy, including intravenous Vincristine™ and oral VP-16™ (Etoposide™), Chlorambucil™ and Prednisone™.

Patient 3 was a 24-year-old housewife who was recently diagnosed as having Hodgkin's lymphoma and commenced on her first cycle of chemotherapy, including intravenous Vincristine™ and oral Chlorambucil™, Procarbazine™, and Prednisone™.

Patient 4 was a 53-year-old male business manager. After a 4-year history of chronic lymphocytic leukemia, he was on his fourth cycle of chemotherapy with oral Chlorambucil™ and Prednisone™, but only the first one that included intravenous drugs, in this case, Vincristine™.

Patient 5 was a 72-year-old male retired engineer. He was diagnosed as having Hodgkin's lymphoma following surgery for intestinal obstruction 3 months previously and was on his first cycle of chemotherapy, including intravenous Vinblastine™ and oral Chlorambucil™, Procarbazine™ and Prednisone™.

Patient 6 was a 46-year-old business woman. She first noticed a lump in her breast some 4 months earlier but did not seek medical attention until the lump had changed and become larger in size. Following diagnosis of breast cancer, she had a mastectomy and removal of axillary lymph nodes. Four weeks after surgery, she commenced on a chemotherapy regimen of intravenous Adriamycin™ and Vincristine™ and oral Tamoxifen™ and Prednisone™.

Patient 7 was a 37-year-old male accountant. He was diagnosed as having Hodgkin's lymphoma 6 weeks earlier and was about to commence on chemotherapy, including intravenous Vinblastine™ and oral Procarbazine™ and Prednisone™.

Table A.1 Summary of background data on patients with burns

No.	Gender	Age	Extent of injury
1	Male	27	5% burns
2	Male	31	5% burns
3	Male	21	25% burns
4	Male	25	12% burns
5	Female	53	6% burns
6	Female	36	15% burns
7	Male	42	25% burns

Table A.2 Summary of background data on patients with cancer

No.	Gender	Age	Medical diagnosis
1	Female	46	Breast carcinoma
2	Female	39	Lymphocytic lymphoma
3	Female	24	Hodgkin's lymphoma
4	Male	53	Chronic lymphocytic leukemia
5	Male	72	Hodgkin's lymphoma
6	Female	46	Breast carcinoma
7	Male	37	Hodgkin's lymphoma

Oncology Clinic and Burn Care Unit nurses

Because there is a lesser amount of individual biographical detail about nurses, data about them are presented only in tabulated form in Tables A.3 and A.4.

Table A.3 Background data on Oncology Clinic (Chemotherapy) nurses

No.	Nursing qualification	Years in nursing practice	Years in Oncology Clinic
1	RegNurse	12.0	0.3
2	RegNurse	13.0	3.0
3	RegNurse	25.0	3.0
4	RegNurse	2.0	0.05

All four Oncology Clinic nurses commented on the stressful nature of their work and a need to balance it with nursing in other settings. During the period of the study, one of the nurses left to return overseas and was hopeful of obtaining work that would not be in the oncology area. Another of the nurses had already taken an 8-month break away from the Oncology Clinic and saw her current involvement as temporary. A third nurse also envisaged staying for no longer than 6 months. Thus, despite the fact that these nurses administered chemotherapy on only one day per week, three of the four expressed a wish to get away from this type of work altogether.

Table A.4 Background data on Burn Care Unit nurses

No.	Nursing qualification	Years in nursing practice	Years in Burn Unit
1	Reg Nurse	9.0	1.5
2	Reg Nurse	7.0	5.0
3	Reg Nurse	4.0	0.2
4	Reg Nurse	5.0	4.5
5	Reg Nurse	12.0	10.0
6	Reg Nurse	1.0	0.5
7	Reg Nurse	10.0	3.0
8	Reg Nurse	3.5	2.5
9	Enr'd Nurse	3.0	2.0
10	Enr'd Nurse	12.0	2.5
11	Reg Nurse	12.0	4.0
12	Enr'd Nurse	7.0	6.0
13	Reg Nurse	11.0	1.5
14	Reg Nurse	13.0	9.0
15	Reg Nurse	8.0	2.0

Overall, nurses working in the Burn Care Unit were young, predominantly in their 20s or early 30s, but with considerable nursing experience. All but one of those who participated in the study had at least 3 years of postregistration nursing experience, the range being from 1 to 13 years, and the mean was 7.8 years. The nursing staff in the Burn Care Unit also showed considerable stability in that all but two had worked there for at least 18 months, the range being from 2.5 months to 10 years, and the mean was 3.6 years. All but one of the nurses interviewed intended to continue working in the unit.

Laboratory nurse

The Laboratory Nurse had 10 years experience in the diagnostic laboratory, mainly in drawing venous blood samples from both hospitalized patients and those attending outpatient clinics. Previously she had worked in a variety of nursing jobs for over 10 years. For Oncology Clinic patients, venepunctures performed in the laboratory emerged as a significant source of inflicted pain, and for this reason, one of the laboratory nurses who frequently performed the venepunctures was observed and interviewed. This is a further example of purposeful sampling used during the study.

Description of the two settings for the study

Clinical settings in which patients with cancer or with burns may be treated can vary a great deal, not only in terms of physical facilities, but also organizationally and in terms of treatment philosophies and protocols. To help the reader understand the context in which the study participants nursed, or were nursed, the two settings are described, and the typical treatments and interventions are outlined.

The Oncology Clinic

This clinic is one of several medical and surgical clinics run as part of a large outpatient department. Patients are referred to the clinic by their family physicians, surgeons, or other specialists. They are assessed and referred for diagnostic tests such as biopsies, radiographic examinations, bone marrow aspirations, or computerized scanning. Once all the information is obtained, the patient and, whenever possible, a family member attend the clinic and are given the diagnosis. An oncologist then discusses with the patient available treatment options and their implications, including the likely side-effects of particular forms of therapy. When chemotherapy is the treatment of choice, patients are asked to attend the Oncology Clinic, which is held every Thursday. During this clinic, the only patients seen are those currently on a chemotherapy protocol of some kind.

Patients can usually choose the time for their appointments, and many do so to fit it in with their work or family commitments. Early morning appointments are preferred since they involve fewer delays and reduce the total amount of time spent at the hospital. It is not uncommon for patients with appointments scheduled for later in the day to spend more than two hours in the clinic for a treatment that may take as little as 15 to 20 minutes. Some patients who are employed may choose late afternoon appointments in order not to cut into their working hours any more than absolutely necessary.

On each visit to the Oncology Clinic, patients first present at the laboratory, where a blood sample is taken for a hematological examination. The larger veins in the intra-cubital fossa (inside aspect of the elbow) are used for this purpose. Patients then wait approximately 10 minutes and are given their test results on a slip of paper, which they take to the Oncology Clinic. Even though the results are openly given to patients, they remain a mystery since the various abbreviations (e.g., WBC for white blood cells) and the related numerical values are not usually explained to them. They do know, however, that a "low blood count" can mean postponement of chemotherapy and further investigations.

On their arrival at the Oncology Clinic, patients hand over the laboratory results to a nurse who usually looks at the results but does not comment on them. The nurse weighs the patient and makes a general inquiry about his or her health and, if not too busy, may talk briefly with the patient and the accompanying person. The patient then waits to be seen by the physician, who will assess the patient's progress, explore any reported problems, consult the laboratory results and decide whether the chemotherapy is to be administered and whether there should be any changes in the medication or dosage. The patient may then have to wait until the nurse has completed her work with another patient. To begin the session, the nurse takes the patient to a treatment room where he or she then has the choice of lying on an examination couch or sitting in an arm chair. In the meantime, the nurse will go away to prepare the medication. Because of the high cost of the drugs used, they are not drawn up in advance but are prepared only after the physician, having seen the patient, decides on the exact medication and dosage. Because of the mode of drug administration, using syringes rather than a continuous infusion from a flask, and the precautionary measures taken, such as wearing gloves and goggles to protect the nurse from the accidental contact with the drugs, the dispensing of cytotoxic and anti-emetic drugs carried out by the nurses can take 10 to 20 minutes, thus further prolonging the waiting time for the patient.

Once the drugs are prepared, the nurse inserts a fine "butterfly" needle (a short, 21 or 23 gauge metal needle with plastic "butterfly" wings used to hold the needle during insertion and to secure it to the patient's skin during the administration of intravenous drugs) into one of the smaller veins on the back of the patient's hand and begins the slow intravenous administration by manually pushing the syringe plunger. The size and fragility of the blood vessels used and the potentially damaging effects of the drugs if extravasation (escape or seepage of blood or injected fluid from a vein into the surrounding tissues or the surface of the skin) occurs mean that the drugs have to be administered very slowly. To reduce possible local tissue damage, cytotoxic drugs are diluted in a saline solution and additional saline solution is used for periodic flushing of the vein. The patients may, therefore, receive 150 mls or more of fluid, delivered in a half dozen or more large syringes and in a 15- to 30-minute period. The majority of patients are also given an intravenous dose of anti-emetic medication to reduce the nausea and vomiting that commonly occur with chemotherapy.

The sedative effects of anti-emetic medication are greater in some patients than in others, but all patients are warned against driving home following chemotherapy and must be accompanied by another person; otherwise, the anti-emetic medication is withheld. Patients are advised to drink at least two liters of fluid on the day of chemotherapy, to eat only light, easily digestible meals, to rest if they find it helpful, and to contact a community health nurse or the hospital oncology ward if any problems such as severe vomiting, pain or other reactions occur. The community health nurse on duty usually telephones patients in the evening of the day on which they had received chemotherapy to ensure that patients are coping and know how to obtain help if necessary.

There is no nursing documentation in relation to the chemotherapy patients apart from a record of the drugs administered and their dosage. Nurses rely on verbal communication with other nurses within and outside the Oncology Clinic and with the physician and resident medical staff. The only documentation is that written by the physician. It is also worth noting that while patients are given detailed verbal explanations of their treatment by the physician they are not given any literature or written information about their disease or treatment other than a Chemotherapy Treatment Card, which lists the drugs they are receiving, lists very brief instructions for the management of symptoms, and provides contact telephone numbers for the community health nurse.

The majority of patients remain on outpatient treatment and are admitted to hospital only if they develop complications. The general atmosphere in the clinic is unhurried, and patients and family members are encouraged to discuss any issues of concern with the physician. The small number of nurses involved with the clinic facilitates continuity of contact, so that over time, patients and nurses come to know each other and share information about social activities and events. Patients are seldom referred to social workers or other support services, but they may be referred to other medical specialists.

The Burn Care Unit

The Burn Care Unit is situated within a 30-bed plastic surgery ward. The number of patients with burns at any one time varies from one or two to 10 or more. The ward caters to all age groups, from young babies to elderly patients. There are isolation facilities for patients whose burns are treated by the exposure method (treatment of burn wounds by leaving them exposed to air) and a large, purpose-built treatment room where saline baths and most of dressing changes are carried out.

The full-time nursing staff include a charge nurse, 12 staff nurses, two enrolled nurses and one nursing aide. In addition, there are eight staff nurses and seven enrolled nurses who work part time, usually 2 to 4 days per week. A patient-assignment mode of nursing care delivery is used, with some attempt to provide continuity of care by assigning a patient to the same nurse on consecutive days. In practice, however, patients do not expect to be nursed by one nurse for more than a day at a time. Enrolled nurses are not assigned to the severely burned patients in the early stages of hospitalization, but they are expected to provide complete care to patients assigned to them, other than the legally proscribed administration of drugs and intravenous fluids.

The ward is served by several surgeons, a senior registrar and two house surgeons (junior medical staff). The lengthy duration of hospitalization and prolonged recovery period experienced by many patients with burns usually has a negative impact on their financial situation, whether the patient is in paid employment at the time of the accident or not. This means that social workers are usually involved with patients and their families from the beginning. Psychologists, on the other hand, are called in only if a patient shows definite and serious signs of psychological disturbance. Some degree of depression, anger, and distress related to painful procedures are accepted by staff as normal and self-limiting, diminishing as the patient's physical condition improves and not requiring interventions other than routine nursing care.

When first admitted to the Burn Care Unit, patients are usually placed in the treatment room and assessed by medical staff. Depending on the severity and extent of the burn injuries, patients may be given intravenous fluids and pain-relieving medication, oxygen therapy, antibiotics, and a tetanus toxoid injection. They are undressed and their burns are cleaned and debrided as much as possible. Patients usually have blood samples taken and may have a catheter inserted into the bladder to facilitate accurate measurement of urinary output and close monitoring of the fluid balance. Patients requiring hospitalization usually have burns that are initially treated by the exposure method. In these cases, patients are placed on sterile bedding and in an isolation room with temperature and humidity controls. Burned areas are swabbed clean with an antiseptic solution every 4 hours, but otherwise, they are left exposed to air. Body parts prone to contractures and needing to be moved, such as hands, are usually smeared with Silver Sulphadiazine™ cream and covered with plastic gloves or plastic wrapping. Once or twice a day, patients are bathed in a saline bath, with any incrustations and cream removed and burned areas debrided and dried. Any visitors to the patient's room are required to wear gowns, masks, and footwear covers.

Burn injuries are not static; rather, they continue to develop over several days. Areas of erythema (superficial redness) and swelling may subside, showing little or no injury, while other areas show necrosis and sloughing as the cells at quite deep levels die from thermal damage. By this time, the patient's condition has usually stabilized, and skin grafting can be considered. Grafting procedures are done in the operating theatre and with the aid of general anaesthesia. Both the donor sites (from which healthy skin is taken for grafting to burned parts of the body) and the grafted areas are covered with sterile dressings, and unless other ungrafted areas remain, patients may be moved out of isolation and into a room with other patients. Graft area dressings are usually left undisturbed for 3 to 4 days and donor site dressings for 8 to 10 days. The initial removal of these dressings can be particularly painful. When there is good healing, and especially with smaller burns, the patient may be allowed to go home at this point, returning daily to the ward clinic for changes of dressings.

Whenever burns are extensive or the graft does not "take" well (i.e., fails to develop adequate blood circulation or becomes infected), additional grafting may be required, and the procedure is repeated. This can extend the patient's time in hospital to many weeks and may be followed by readmissions for further grafting to release contractures and to provide better functional and cosmetic results.

The relatively small number of burn patients in the ward at any one time means that patients seldom have access to someone with similar injuries and at the same stage of recovery with whom they can compare progress and evaluate their own coping. In the absence of such input, patients rely on nurses for feedback on their progress and behavior in the situation.

Ethical considerations

The protocol for the study was submitted to the Massey University Human Ethics Research Committee and to the Research Ethics Committee of the Hospital Board within which the study was to be conducted and their approval was received. Prior to the first interview, participants received a verbal explanation of the study, its purposes, and what would be required of them during the study. Steps taken to ensure confidentiality and anonymity of interview and observational data were explained, and participants' were told they could ask for further information or withdraw from the study at any time. In addition, participants were provided with a written explanation of the study and were asked to sign an informed consent form. All patients were given time to consider their participation and to consult their families if they wished prior to giving their consent. They were also provided with a card giving the researcher's full name, work address and telephone number.

From the outset of the study, it was explained to the participants that the aim of the research was to describe experiences of the patients and nurses as they happen and not to alter them in any way. In that sense, the study posed no risks to the participants' well-being. Nevertheless, I accepted that some patients might find participation in interviews, requiring them to recall painful or unpleasant experiences, distressing. On four occasions when this did occur, the tape recorder was turned off, and an offer was made to terminate the interview. I stayed with the patient, however, and provided emotional support through touch, use of silence, and verbal assurances that expression of one's feelings is a normal and necessary part of healing. In each case the patients, after a time, requested that the interview continue and expressed a sense of relief in having been able to cry and openly share their distress in a supportive atmosphere.

I also adopted the stance that informed consent involves more than signing a statement at the beginning of a study and that it is an ongoing process of negotiation throughout the period of data collection. Decisions about the timing and location of each interview and my assurances to the participants indicating that they were free to choose which questions they would answer and in how much detail were all seen as part of the ongoing consent negotiation.

In line with the assurances provided to the research ethics committees and study participants, all data for the study were collected by me, code numbers and pseudonyms were used on data transcripts, and interview tapes were erased on completion of the study.

INVESTIGATING THE EXPERIENCE OF INFLICTED PAIN AS IT IS LIVED: METHODS OF DATA COLLECTION

As discussed at some length in Chapter 1 and mentioned again in Chapter 2, the experience of pain, and especially so of inflicted pain, has received very limited attention in the research and other professional literature. Scarry (1985) notes that even artistic and literary representations of bodily pain are difficult to find. While depictions of suffering are common and lie at the heart of great literature, from Tolstoy (1918/1973) and Tagore (1916/1985) to women writers like Angelou (1984) and little known immigrant writers like Skrzynecki (1987), pain is different. Confronted with bodily pain "even the artist—whose lifework and everyday habit are to refine and extend the reflexes of speech—ordinarily falls silent before pain" (Scarry, 1985, p. 10).

However rare research and literary representations of the experience of pain might be, as a nurse I knew that I could turn to "the experts" (Swanson-Kauffman & Schonwald, 1988), that is, patients and nurses who live with the reality of inflicted pain on a daily basis. The clinical setting also promised a possibility for understanding the context in which pain is inflicted and endured: a key factor given that "to understand a person's behavior or expressions, one has to study the person in context, for it is only there that what a person values and finds significant is visible" (Leonard, 1989, p. 46). A number of specific procedures were used within the general field study design to obtain information from patients and nurses that constituted the text for analysis and description.

Participant observation and recording

Throughout the 5 months of data collection, from November 1987 to April 1988, I (as the sole researcher) participated in the life of the Oncology Clinic and the Burn Care Unit. This involved being present during staff meetings, especially during staff hand-over reports, sitting in on medical and nursing consultations with patients, attending medical rounds, and assisting nurses in their work when a second pair of hands was needed, such as when preparing or tidying up the treatment rooms, moving bed-bound patients, or opening packs of sterile equipment needed during a procedure.

In addition, I was present as an observer during at least three procedures (such as dressing changes or administration of intravenous chemotherapy) conducted with each patient who participated in the study. Such procedures could last from a few minutes to over 2 hours. Field notes were recorded both during and after each period of observation and related to the nature of the procedure; the preparation received by the patient, including explanations about possible pain and any analgesic medication given; the nurse's and patient's verbal and nonverbal behaviors and interactions with each other; the duration of the procedure; and its overall impact on the patient and the nurse or nurses involved.

Patient interviews

Following the patient's experience of a procedure that carried some potential for being painful, each patient participated in a semistructured interview, which focused on the experience of the procedure and any associated pain. At least three interviews were completed with each patient, the initial one also including biographical information, past health history, and experience of the current illness or injury. The last interview was usually conducted close to the time of discharge or completion of a therapy cycle and was used to generate new information as well as to review previous observations and validate some of the emerging conceptual categories and themes.

In all, 48 interviews were completed with the 14 patients in the study, varying in duration from 15 to 90 minutes. All interviews were tape recorded and transcribed for detailed analysis. The interviews took the form of free-flowing dialogue, usually triggered by requests such as "In your own words, tell me about having the chemotherapy [or your dressings changed] this morning." Observations made during a procedure were explored and clarified during interviews through comments or questions such as "You seemed to give a big sigh when the dressing had finally come off; tell me what you were feeling at that time," or "When the nurse missed getting the needle in the first time, what were your thoughts at that time?" During interviews patients were also asked to rate the intensity of the pain they had experienced in the course of a particular procedure. A 10-point verbal rating scale was used, where zero indicated "no pain" and 10 indicated "the worst possible pain." (Initial plans to use a visual analogue scale were abandoned because of the problems associated with the use of pen and paper by patients with burn injuries.)

Interviews were conducted after the completion of a period of observation, sometimes immediately after; but whenever the patient was tired or expressed preference for a delay, the interview was conducted at a time most suitable for the patient. In the Burns Care Unit that sometimes meant that a patient would rest or sleep following a lengthy bathing and dressing change procedure, and the interview would be conducted later in the day. Interviews took place in patients' rooms, which meant private single rooms initially but shared rooms during the latter part of hospitalization. While shared rooms presented some problems related to privacy, the technical difficulties in carrying out the interviews were a greater problem, with more frequent interruptions and extraneous noise from other patients' conversations, radio and television sets.

Interviews with the oncology patients were conducted on completion of chemotherapy in the privacy of a clinic room set aside for the interviews or, in the case of two patients and at their request, in the patient's own home. Accommodating to patient preferences was an important part of maintaining rapport with the participants, especially the oncology patients. Some of them found visits to the clinic very stressful and felt a strong need to leave the hospital as soon as their therapy was completed. Once in their own home, however, they talked freely about their experience.

The potential for adding to patients' suffering through the need to have them relive painful and distressing experiences during research interviews was offset by the potential for therapeutic release within each interview. Patients found it helpful to tell their story, to discuss their experiences and thus gain a sense of order and meaning in what had initially seemed a confusing set of events or experiences. Patients with cancer especially used the interviews to validate their subjective experiences, such as pervasive feelings of tiredness, as real and common to other patients receiving chemotherapy. In the absence of contact with other people with cancer, the research interviews provided these patients with therapeutic opportunities to express their thoughts and feelings and to seek validation of their experiences.

Nurse interviews

Interviews with nurses were conducted after their participation in a treatment procedure on a patient included in the study. Most often they took place at the end of a shift, that is, in the afternoons or late evenings. Having completed their work for the day, nurses were able to set aside 20 to 40 minutes needed for each interview. All interviews with nurses were conducted in a closed office, ensuring privacy and good technical quality of tape recording, although even these interviews were not without interruptions.

A total of 41 nurse interviews were completed, the number of interviews with individual nurses ranging from one to five and depending primarily on the level of their involvement in the care of the patients included in the study.

During the first part of the initial interview, each nurse was asked to provide information about her nursing qualifications and experience and her views about the general needs of the patients with whom she worked. This was followed by the more focused inquiry into the nature of the procedures performed on patients as part of nurses' work in the particular setting and the discussion about the specific procedure performed by the nurse earlier that day. Nurses were asked to comment on how much contact they had with a particular patient prior to that day and whether or not they had performed any procedures on that particular patient previously. A discussion of the nurse's experience of a specific procedure usually began with a statement such as "Take me through the process of Mr X's dressing change this morning, right from when you were told that you would be looking after him today," or "Tell me what it was like to give Mrs Y her chemotherapy today." Participants' comments were explored and clarified, and particular aspects of the procedure observed by the researcher discussed: for example, why an oncology patient was asked or not asked to place hands in a basin of warm water prior to the insertion of the intravenous needle on a given occasion.

Two specific questions were asked of most participants, their timing usually guided by the issues raised in the discussion: "What can you do to make the procedure less painful for the patient?" and "What can you do to make the procedure less stressful for yourself?" These questions emerged only after initial interviews during which the painfulness of the procedures and the stressfulness of the nurses' work began to appear as important themes.

As with the interviews with the patients, all 41 interviews with nurses were audiotaped and transcribed for detailed analysis.

Review of patients' records

A review of the nursing and medical records relating to the patients included in the study was undertaken, with a particular focus on the documentation of pain assessment and management, drugs prescribed and administered, and patients' coping with their illness and with the painful procedures. While nurses in the Burn Care Unit produced nursing care plans and kept daily records of the patients' progress, there were no nursing records kept by the nurses in the Oncology Clinic other than the documentation of the drugs administered on each occasion.

Information extracted from patients' records formed a specific section of the field notes and thus became part of the text for data analysis. Use of written patient records also allowed for "triangulation" of data sources, thus contributing to a clearer understanding of the patients' and nurses' experiences, especially in relation to medication for pain relief. The purpose of data source triangulation, of drawing on different sources of data and relating them to each other, is to overcome possible deficiencies in any one data source and "to maximize the range of data that might contribute to a more complete understanding of the topic being investigated" (Knafl & Breitmayer, 1991).

REFLECTING ON THE ESSENTIAL THEMES THAT EMERGED FROM THE INVESTIGATION: METHODS OF DATA ANALYSIS AND INTERPRETATION

As data collection proceeds and the researcher begins to accumulate field notes and interview transcripts, the raw data need to be managed and analyzed. Data management involves the practical tasks of collection, coding, storage, and retrieval of materials. Data analysis, on the other hand, involves reading the data texts, reflecting on the whole and parts of data, producing conceptual classifications of data, and creating conceptual memos, such as commentaries, insights, and questions for further consideration (Ammon-Gaberson & Piantanida, 1988; Knafl & Webster, 1988; Lynch-Sauer, 1985).

In the present study, data management involved having transcriptions made of all interviews and field notes and manually sorting all the textual material into groupings related to the four categories of participants: the Oncology Clinic patients and nurses and the Burn Care Unit patients and nurses. In addition, colored markers, margin comments, and cut and paste methods were used later to identify and retrieve information dealing with particular categories of data.

The conceptual processes of data analysis are more difficult to describe in an orderly fashion. This is because the activities and transformations involved did not always occur in a tidy chronological sequence. Rather, the processes both overlapped and were repeated as more data accumulated and new insights were gained. In line with the phenomenological approach, field notes, interview transcripts, and extracts from patients' records constituted the text for thematic analysis (Benner, 1985; van Manen, 1990). At all stages of analysis and interpretation attempts were made to preserve the close link with the original data of the patients' and nurses' experience. One way in which this was done involved returning to the original tape recordings to clarify or confirm the presence of pauses, silences, tone of voice, emphasis, intonation, and other paralinguistic aspects of the interview data.

The use of concurrent data collection and early reading of whole interviews allowed for comparative shifts between the emerging whole and the accounts of specific experiences, and this constituted the first phase of interpretation. This, in turn, provided additional questions for ongoing data collection. For example, it was the early reading of the nurses' interviews that suggested stressfulness of inflicting pain as a significant aspect of nurses' work, especially in the Burn Care Unit. As "an aspect of the structure of lived experience" this then emerged as a theme (van Manen, 1990, p. 87). The meaning of this theme was explored through later, more detailed analysis and ongoing reflection.

Another phase of the analysis involved reading all interview transcripts and field notes to obtain a general sense of the data as a whole, the range of issues raised by the participants, and the boundaries and scope of the study, from its initial aims to what it could be seen to have accomplished. As Benner (1985) suggests, "Whole cases can be compared to whole cases" (p. 9), thus revealing new issues or themes. It was through the reading of whole interviews and through attentiveness to what they revealed about the person in each case that I was alerted to the contextual significance of the changed body for the patients. At the same time, it became apparent that the reality of the changed body was a very different issue for nurses.

Following this phase, a detailed, line-by-line analysis of all transcripts was undertaken, identifying significant statements pertaining to the phenomenon of inflicted pain and the context in which it is experienced. These statements were extracted from all data sources and examined for similarities, complementary aspects and conflicting points of view. The interpretive (hermeneutic) approach to this material resulted in the identification of category clusters and themes as they related to the patients' experience of inflicted pain in two quite different settings and to the nurses' experience of contributing to patients' pain. The thematic analysis, using a detailed line-by-line approach, was used to isolate "thematic statements" (van Manen, 1990), which were interpreted further through reflection and dialogue with the data.

Analysis is not only a matter of identifying data that pertain to the topic of the study. A phenomenological description of pain, or any other phenomenon in which personal experience is transformed into a systematic written account, involves interpretation, both on the part of those describing the experience and the researcher studying the phenomenon. Hermeneutic phenomenology, according to van Manen (1990), attends to two issues simultaneously: it stays close to the original data and describes things as they appear, and it interprets that which it observes since "there are no such things as uninterpreted phenomena" (p. 180). Put differently, people who are hurting experience pain in a direct, embodied way, but the phenomenon of pain that the researcher presents is something created through interpretation of the participants' and the researcher's understandings of what it means to experience pain. Hermeneutics, as "the theory and practice of interpretation" (van Manen, 1990, p. 179), has long been used in the analysis of historical texts within their cultural, historical, and literary contexts (Lundin,

Thiselton, & Walhout, 1985) and has only more recently been employed in interpretive nursing research (Benner, 1984a, 1985; Lionberger, 1985). The task, according to Benner (1985), is to "uncover the meanings in everyday practice in such a way that they are not destroyed, distorted, decontextualized, trivialized, or sentimentalized" (p. 6). Instead, the findings of phenomenological research can be presented in a way that deepens understanding in context and keeps the findings close to the lived experience.

In the present study, return to original transcripts permitted identification of extracts and exemplar cases that best capture the essence of particular themes. In line with the hermeneutic approach, exemplars are therefore used extensively to present the findings and keep them close to the original data and to allow the reader to participate in the process of consensual validation (Benner, 1985; Leonard, 1989).

Throughout all phases of the study, I also kept a written log of interpretive comments and questions, which arose out of my background knowledge, the experience of being involved in the research and the lifeworld of study participants, and the reflections on that experience. These "memos" constituted important personal insights into the nature of the participants' experience and its meaning.

In addition, interpretations made from individual participant's data, as well as grouped data, were validated whenever possible in the final interviews with each participant. Nurses in both settings also participated in a final group discussion designed to facilitate validation of the preliminary findings. These group discussions were of particular importance in relation to the nurses in the Burn Care Unit where it was not always possible to predict which individual interview would be the last one for a particular nurse.

While every attempt was made to treat the data and each phase of the research process with honesty and integrity, the final interpretation reflects the researcher's intimate involvement in the process of transformation of the experience of others into public knowledge. While another researcher, adopting a different perspective, may have arrived at a different interpretation of the phenomenon, it is my contention that the findings presented in this report constitute a valid interpretation of the experience of clinically inflicted pain.

DESCRIBING THE PHENOMENON AND BRINGING IT TO SPEECH: PRESENTATION OF FINDINGS

In presenting the results of a phenomenological study, there is a need to keep the final description close to the original data (Benner, 1985) and true to the inner intent and meaning carried within the data. As van Manen (1984) has pointed out,

> Phenomenological research is a poetizing activity....And that is why, when you listen to a presentation of a phenomenological nature, you will listen in vain for the punchline, the latest information, or the big news. As in poetry, it is inappropriate to ask for a conclusion or a summary of a phenomenological study. To summarize a poem in order to present the result would destroy the result because the poem is the result. (p. 2)

A number of different approaches can be adopted to structure the presentation of phenomenological research. Van Manen (1990, pp. 167–173) identifies at least five possible ways of textual organization: *thematic, analytical, exemplificative, exegetical,* and *existential.* Van Manen suggests that the list is neither exhaustive, nor are the five approaches mutually exclusive. The main approach adopted for the presentation of the findings is thematic, whereby the focal meanings of the experience of inflicted pain are captured and used to describe the structure of that experience. Themes are a means of "getting at the meaning of the experience," of expressing the essence of the phenomenon, and of "giving shape" to human experience that nevertheless retains an element of the unshareable (van Manen, 1990, p. 88). To the extent that the comparisons are made between the experiences of patients with cancer and those with burn injuries, the text is also organized exemplificatively, varying the examples of pain experience in order to deepen the understanding of the phenomenon of clinically inflicted pain.

ENDNOTE

[1]Literature dealing with children's pain, its assessment and management is dominated by developmental considerations and theories. Inclusion of children in this study would have necessitated a review of a much wider area of literature and adjustments to data collection methods and procedures.

Appendix B
Glossary of Technical Terms

Acupan™ (nefopam hydrocloride): A nonopioid analgesic used in the treatment of acute pain. The mechanism of its action is unknown. Side-effects include nausea, dizziness, drowsiness, and dry mouth.

Adjuvant drugs. Drugs given as a secondary remedy to assist the action of other primary drugs or other forms of therapy.

Adriamycin™ (doxorubicin hydrochloride): An antitumor antibiotic that destroys cancer cells by interfering with nucleic acid synthesis. Common side-effects include bone marrow suppression, loss of body hair, and stomatitis (inflammation of the mouth, with or without ulceration).

Analgesic Drugs: Drugs that relieve pain.

Angiography: A radiological examination of blood vessels following an injection of a radio-opaque dye.

Arterial puncture: Insertion of a needle into an artery, usually to obtain a blood specimen. The puncture is usually made into the femoral artery in the groin area.

Arteriography: A radiological examination of arteries following an injection of a radio-opaque dye.

Aseptic necrosis of bone: Death or loss of bone tissue in the absence of microorganisms, often leading to bone fractures. May be caused by high doses of corticosteroid hormones used in the treatment of cancer.

Aspirin (acetylsalicylic acid): An analgesic and anti-inflammatory drug that acts locally by inhibiting prostaglandin synthesis. It also reduces fever and delays blood clotting. Side-effects include nausea and epigastric burning, with high risk of gastro-intestinal hemorrhage in patients with bleeding disorders, history of peptic ulcers, those at risk of developing stress ulcers (including patients with severe burns), and the elderly.

Cachexia: A condition of extreme debility, characterized by severe emaciation, weakness and anemia and usually seen in the terminal phase of cancer.

Causalgia: An intense burning pain that persists following trauma to a peripheral nerve.

Chlorambucil (leukeran™): A cytotoxic drug, derivative of nitrogen mustard. Like other alkylating agents, it acts to destroy cancer cells by producing highly reactive ions that bind to particular (e.g., DNA) molecules within cells. Side-effects include bone marrow suppression, nausea and vomiting (less frequent when drug is given orally).

Chronic lymphocytic leukemia: A malignant disease of the blood cells in which there is a proliferation of white blood cells and enlargement of the lymphatic glands and the spleen.

Codeine (codeine phosphate): An opioid analgesic used alone or in combination with other pain-relieving drugs such as aspirin or acetaminophen (paracetamol) to relieve mild to moderate pain. Side-effects include constipation, nausea, dizziness, and drowsiness.

Cytotoxyc drugs: A range of anticancer drugs which interfere with cell structures and/or cell division.

Deafferentation pain: Pain (often of a burning quality) that follows upon damage to the sensory nerve pathways that normally transmit nociceptive information.

Debridement: Removal of foreign substances and injured tissues from burn or other traumatic wounds in order to remove potential sources of infection and to promote healing.

Diazepam (Valium™): One of the benzodiazepine group of drugs. Used as a tranquilizer, sedative, skeletal muscle relaxant, and anticonvulsant.

Enrolled nurse: A nurse who has undergone an 18-month (or more recently a 12-month) education program based in a hospital school of nursing. Enrolled nurses must work under the supervision of a registered nurse or physician.

Epistemology: Part of philosophy concerned with theories of knowledge, particularly how knowledge is acquired and validated.

Extravasation: The leakage of injection solution out of a vein and into surrounding tissues; a possible complication of intravenous chemotherapy. When extravasated *irritant* anticancer drugs (e.g., VP-16) may cause inflammation, increased pigmentation, and burning sensation. *Vesicant* anticancer drugs (e.g., Adriamycin, Vincristine) may cause severe ulceration and necrosis of local tissues, which may require surgical excision and skin grafting).

Fibrosis: Formation of fibrous tissue as in scars, sometimes due to inflammation caused by radiotherapy.

Fortral™ (pentazocine): A narcotic analgesic used in the treatment of moderate to severe acute pain. Side-effects include nausea, vomiting, dizziness, sedation, euphoria, as well as headaches and hallucinations in some patients.

Hodgkin's lymphoma (Hodgkin's disease): A malignant disease affecting lymphocytes (white blood cells formed in the lymphoid tissue) and characterized by an enlargement of lymph nodes, fatigue, and general malaise. (Distinguished from other types of lymphomas by the presence of the multinucleated Reed-Sternberg giant cell on histological examination.)

Iatrogenic: A condition caused by medical examination or treatment.

IM (intramuscular): An injection of medication into a muscle, e.g., the deltoid in the upper arm or the gluteal in the buttock.

Intrathecal: Placement of a needle or injection between the membranes of the spinal cord, usually in the subarachnoid space.

IV (intravenous): An injection of medication (or infusion of fluid) into a vein.

Laparotomy: Opening of the abdomen by surgical incision for exploratory purposes.

Lymphangiography: A radiological examination of lymph vessels following an injection of a radio-opaque dye.

Lymphocytic lymphoma: (A form of Non-Hodgkin's lymphoma) A malignant disease of the lymphoid tissue, similar in manifestation to Hodgkin's disease but with a different clinical course, prognosis and treatment.

Lymphoedema: Swelling of the arm and hand as a result of the accumulation of lymph (fluid) in the tissues, usually due to the obstruction of lymph drainage through the lymph nodes in the axilla.

Lymphoma: A tumor of lymphoid tissue.

Mammography: An X-ray examination of the breast for presence of tumors.

Maxolon™ (metoclopramide hydrochloride): An anti-emetic drug used to control nausea and vomiting commonly seen with chemotherapy administration. Maxolon also acts as a sedative.

Metastasis: Transference of tumor cells from primary growth to other organs or parts of the body.

Metastatic disease: Disease related to the spread of a primary tumor to other parts of the body, usually through blood or lymph vessels.

Meperidine (Demerol™): See Pethidine.

Morphine (morphine sulphate): An alkaloid derivative of opium, which acts in the central nervous system. Widely used in the treatment of severe acute pain.

Naproxen (Naprosyn™): A nonsteroidal anti-inflammatory drug used in the treatment of pain, particularly that accompanied by inflammation. Side-effects include abdominal discomfort, headache, nausea, vertigo, and peripheral swelling.

Needle aspiration: Withdrawal of fluid from a cyst or a body cavity through a hollow needle.

Needle biopsy: Insertion of a hollow needle through the skin and other overlying tissues for the purpose of withdrawing a small specimen of tissue for laboratory analysis. Commonly used in biopsy of breast tumors.

Neoplastic disease: Disease related to new and abnormal growth of tissue, usually a tumor, in some part of the body.

Neurodestructive procedures: Severing or destruction of nerve pathways, usually by surgery, in order to control pain.

Nociception: Response of sensory nerves to a noxious stimulus (i.e., a stimulus capable of producing tissue damage) or to one that would become noxious if prolonged.

Oncology: Branch of medicine specializing in the study and treatment of tumors, i.e., cancer.

Ontology: Part of philosophy dealing with nature of being.

Panadeine™: A combination of Paracetamol™ (acetaminophen) and codeine, which provides more effective pain relief than provided by either drug administered alone. Used in the treatment of moderate to severe pain. Side-effects are mainly those of codeine (constipation, nausea, dizziness, and drowsiness).

Panadol™: See Paracetamol™.

Pancreatitis: Inflammation of the pancreas, a gland lying behind the stomach. In acute inflammation, pancreatic enzymes can cause self-digestion, which is accompanied by severe pain.

Paracetamol™ (acetaminophen, Panadol™): A mild oral analgesic that also reduces fever but (unlike aspirin) has minimal anti-inflammatory effect. Used in treatment of headache and common musculoskeletal pains. Side-effects are uncommon with therapeutic doses, but potentially fatal liver damage follows serious overdosage.

Patient Controlled Analgesia: Intermittent and/or continuous intravenous infusion of pain-relieving medication with inbuilt mechanism for patients to self-administer incremental doses according to need (but within preset safety limits).

Percutaneous transhepatic cholangiography: A radiological examination of the gall bladder and bile ducts following the injection of a radio-opaque dye through the chest or abdominal wall and the liver.

Pethidine (pethidine hydrochloride): An opiate analgesic drug used in the treatment of moderate to severe pain. Its most distinctive feature is its short duration of action (2–3 hours). (Known as meperidine or demerol in USA.)

Prednisone (Delta-Cortelan™): A corticosteroid hormone used to suppress tumor growth as an adjuvant to other cytotoxic chemotherapy. Side-effects include appetite stimulation, sleep disturbances, mood arousal and euphoria. Corticosteroids can mask infections and peptic ulceration and contribute to osteoporosis.

Primary nursing: A system of nursing care delivery where one (primary) nurse takes responsibility for patient assessment, planning of care, implementation of care whenever on duty, and ongoing evaluation of patient's progress and responses to nursing interventions. In the absence of the primary nurse, care is provided by other (associate) nurses on the basis of established care plans. The system offers greater continuity of care and, potentially, more individualized care.

Procarbazine hydrochloride (Natulan™, Mutalane™): A cytotoxic drug, possibly with alkylating properties, used particularly in Hodgkin's lymphoma. Side-effects include reduction in blood cells, including platelets, and nausea and vomiting, the latter being more common at the onset of treatment.

Psychotropic drugs: Drugs that affect the mind or alter mood, including anti-depressants, tranquilizers, and sedatives.

Registered nurse (comprehensive): A nurse who has completed a 3-year education program in a polytechnic or a technical institute school of nursing. Qualified to work in any field of nursing, except midwifery.

Registered nurse (general): A nurse who has completed a 3-year education program in a hospital-based school of nursing. Qualified to work in community and general hospital settings but requiring further education to work in the psychiatric or psychopaedic areas or as a midwife.

Savlon™ (chlorhexidine gluconate 1.5% and cetrimide 15%): An antiseptic and cleansing solution used in swabbing burns and other wounds.

Silver sulphadiazine: A topical antibiotic cream used to prevent and treat wound infection in severe burns. Particularly effective against Gram-negative organisms such as *Pseudomonas aeruginosa*. Usually combined with chlorhexidine digluconate (Silvazine™).

Tamoxifen (Tamofen™, Genox™): Anti-oestrogenic hormone used to suppress tumor growth, particularly in breast cancer. Side-effects include "hot flashes," dizziness, nausea and vomiting.

Valium™: See Diazepam.

Venepuncture: Insertion of a needle into a vein, usually to obtain a blood specimen.

Vinblastine sulphate (Velbe™, Velban™): A plant alkaloid derived from the periwinkle (*Vinca rosea*). It destroys cancer cells by crystallizing certain proteins within them and arresting cell division. Side-effects include bone marrow depression and resulting reduction in white blood cells, nausea and vomiting, loss of body hair, stomatitis (inflammation of the mouth), and ulceration of local tissue if drug leaks or is spilled on the skin.

Vincristine sulphate (Oncovin™): A plant alkaloid derived from the periwinkle (*Vinca rosea*). Acts in similar fashion to vinblastine. Side-effects include neurotoxicity with ensuing peripheral numbness, weakness, cranial nerve palsies, vocal cord paralysis, urinary retention, constipation, and paralytic ileus (a form of bowel obstruction). Severe ulceration and necrosis may follow leakage or spillage of the drug on the skin.

VP-16 (Etoposide™): A plant alkaloid, used in treatment of cancer, similar in action to vinblastine. Side-effects include suppression of white blood cells and platelets, loss of body hair, anorexia, nausea and vomiting.

REFERENCES

Allen R. E. (Ed.). (1990). *The concise Oxford dictionary of current English* (8th ed.). Oxford: Clarendon Press.

Cape, B. F. (1968). *Bailliere's nurses' dictionary* (17th ed.). London: Bailliere, Tindall and Cassell.

Fields, H. L. (1987). *Pain.* New York: McGraw-Hill Book Company.

Groenwald, S. L. (1987). *Cancer nursing: Principles and practices.* Boston: Jones and Bartlett Publishers.

Heel, R. C. (Ed.). (1988). *New ethicals catalogue, 25*(3). Auckland: ADIS Press.

Powers, B. A., & Knapp, T. R. (1990). *A Dictionary of nursing theory and research.* London: Sage Publications.

Schmidt, R. (Ed.). (1988). *New ethicals compendium.* Auckland: ADIS Press.

Speight, T. M. (Ed.). (1989). *Therapeutic drug index, 2*(1). Auckland: The Medical Publishing Co.

Wall, P. D., & Melzack, R. (Eds.). (1989). *Textbook of pain* (2nd ed.). Edinburgh: Churchill Livingstone.

Bibliography

Abu-Saad, H. (1984). Assessing children's responses to pain. *Pain, 19,* 163–171.

Addis, L. (1986). Pains and other secondary mental entities. *Philosophy and Phenomenological Research, 47*(1), 59–73.

Adelman, S. (1984). Mr Cohen and the headache. *Journal of the American Medical Association, 251*(9), 1168.

Ahles, T. A., Blanchard, E. B., & Ruckdeschel, J. C. (1983). The multi-dimensional nature of cancer-related pain. *Pain, 17,* 277–288.

Ahles, T. A., Ruckdeschel, J. C., & Blanchard, E. B. (1984). Cancer-related pain—1. Prevalence in an outpatient setting as a function of stage of disease and type of cancer. *Journal of Psychosomatic Research, 28*(2), 115–119.

Ammon-Gaberson, K. B., & Piantanida, M. (1988). Generating results from qualitative data. *Image, 20*(3), 159–161.

Anderson, J. M. (1989). The phenomenological perspective. In J. M. Morse (Ed.), *Qualitative nursing research: A contemporary dialogue* (pp. 15–26). Rockville, MD: Aspen Publishers.

Angarola, R. T. (1986). Narcotic analgesics: Fears and responsibilities. *Journal of Pain and Symptom Management, 1*(2), 77–78.

Angelou, M. (1984). *I know why the caged bird sings*. London: Virago Press.

Angus, J. E., & Faux, S. (1989). The effects of music on adult postoperative patients' pain during a nursing procedure, In S. G. Funk, E. M. Tornquist, M. T. Champagne, L. A. Copp, & R. A. Wiese (Eds.), *Key aspects of comfort: Management of pain, fatigue, and nausea* (pp. 166–172). New York: Springer Publishing Company.

Anton, M. -C. (1984). Caught in the webb: A nurse's experience. *Medicine and Human Rights, 7*(January), 1–2.

Atchison, N., Guercio, P., & Monaco, C. (1986). Pain in the pediatric burn patient: Nursing assessment and perception. *Issues in Comprehensive Pediatric Nursing, 9*, 399–409.

Barkas, G., & Duafala, M. E. (1988). Advances in cancer pain management: A review of patient-controlled analgesia. *Journal of Pain and Symptom Management, 3*(3), 150–160.

Barratt, D. (1988). Seeing darkly: Some thoughts on how we know and how much. *Christian Arena, 41*(1), 6–9.

Bayley, E. W. (1990). Wound healing in the patient with burns. *Nursing Clinics of North America, 25*(1), 205–222.

Bench, R. J. (1989). Health science, natural science, and clinical knowledge. *Journal of Medicine and Philosophy, 14*, 147–164.

Benner, P. (1984a). *From novice to expert: Excellence and power in clinical nursing practice*. Menlo Park, CA: Addison-Wesley.

Benner, P. (1984b). *Stress and satisfaction on the job*. New York: Praeger Scientific Press.

Benner, P. (1985). Quality of life: A phenomenological perspective on explanation, prediction, and understanding in nursing science. *Advances in Nursing Science, 8*(1), 1–14.

Benner, P., & Tanner, C. (1987). Clinical judgement: How expert nurses use intuition. *American Journal of Nursing, 87,* 23.

Benner, P., & Wrubel, J. (1989). *The primacy of caring: Stress and coping in health and illness.* Menlo Park, CA: Addison-Wesley.

Bergum, V. (1989). Being a phenomenological researcher. In J. M. Morse (Ed.), *Qualitative nursing research: A contemporary dialogue* (pp. 43–57). Rockville, MD: Aspen Publishers.

Bernard, V. W., Ottenberg, P., & Redl, F. (1977). Dehumanization: A composite psychological defense in relation to modern war. In A. Monat & R. S. Lazarus (Eds.), *Stress and coping: An anthology* (pp. 285–306). New York: Columbia University Press, .

Beyer, J. E., De Good, D. E., Ashley, L. C., & Russell, G. A. (1983). Patterns of postoperative analgesic use with adults and children following cardiac surgery. *Pain, 17,* 71–81.

Bishop, A. H., & Scudder, J. R. (1990). *The practical, moral, and personal sense of nursing.* Albany, NY: State University of New York Press

Blotcky, A. D. (1986). Helping adolescents with cancer cope with their disease. *Seminars in Oncology Nursing, 2*(2), 117–122.

Bologh, R. W. (1981). Grounding the alienation of self and body: A critical, phenomenological analysis of the patient in Western medicine. *Sociology of Health and Illness, 3*(2), 188–206.

Bond, M. R. (1981). Patients' experience of pain. *Pharmacology and Therapeutics, 12,* 563–573.

Bonica, J. J. (1980). Pain research and therapy: Past and current status and future needs. In L. K. Y. Ng & J. J. Bonica (Eds.), *Pain, discomfort and humanitarian care* (pp. 1–46). New York: Elsevier North Holland.

Brink, P. J. (1991). Issues of reliability and validity. In J. M. Morse (Ed.), *Qualitative nursing research: A contemporary dialogue* (Rev. ed. pp. 164–186). Newbury Park, CA: Sage Publications.

Brown, L. (1986). The experience of care: Patient perspectives. *Topics in Clinical Nursing, 8*(2), 56–62.

Bryan-Brown, C. W. (1986). Development of pain management in critical care. In M. J. Cousins & G. D. Phillips (Eds.), *Acute pain management* (pp. 1–19). New York: Churchill Livingstone.

Campbell, K. (1984). *Body and mind* (2nd ed.). Notre Dame, ID: University of Notre Dame Press.

Campbell, S. H. (1986). The meaning of breast cancer/mastectomy experience. *Humane Medicine, 2*(2), 91–95.

Cason, J. S. (1981). *Treatment of burns.* London: Chapman and Hall.

Caton, D. (1985). The secularization of pain. *Anesthesiology, 62,* 493–501.

Chapman, C. R. (1988). Pain related to cancer treatment. *Journal of Pain and Symptom Management, 3*(4), 188–193.

Chapman, C. R., Syrjala, K., & Sargur, M. (1985). Pain as a manifestation of cancer treatment. *Seminars in Oncology Nursing, 1*(2), 100–108.

Chisolm, D (1987). From the heart: A biography of Sir Brian Barratt-Boyes. *Metro, 7*(77), 72–93.

Choiniere, M., Melzack, R., Rondeau, J., Girard, N., & Paquin, M. -J. (1989). The pain of burns: Characteristics and correlates. *The Journal of Trauma, 29*(11), 1531–1539.

Christensen, J. C. (1988). *The nursed passage: A theoretical framework for the nurse-patient partnership.* Unpublished doctoral dissertation, Massey University, Palmerston North, New Zealand.

Coates, M. B. (1986). Distress caused by urethral catheters. *Anaesthesia, 41*(6), 670.

Cohen, A. (1984). Descartes, consciousness and depersonalization: Viewing the history of philosophy from a Strausian perspective. *Journal of Medicine and Philosophy, 9*(1), 7–27.

Cohen, M. Z. (1987). A historical overview of the phenomenological movement. *Image, 19*(1), 31–34.

Colaizzi, P. F. (1978). Psychological research as the phenomenologist views it. In R. S. Valle & M. King (Eds.), *Existential-phenomenological alternatives for psychology* (pp. 48–71). New York: Oxford University Press.

Copp, L. A. (1985). Pain, ethics and the negotiation of values. In L. A. Copp (Ed.), *Perspectives on pain* (pp. 137–150). Edinburgh: Churchill Livingstone.

Coyle, N. (1985). Symptom management: Pain—an overview of current concepts. *Cancer Nursing, 8*(Suppl. 1), 44–49.

Coyle, N., & Foley, K. (1985). Pain in patients with cancer: Profile of patients and common pain syndromes. *Seminars in Oncology Nursing, 1*(2), 93–99.

David, C. (1982). Work on a burn unit and plastic surgery ward during the Yom Kippur War. In N. A. Milgram (Ed.), *Stress and anxiety* (Vol. 8, pp. 389–396). Washington, DC: Hemisphere Pub. Corp.

De Moulin, D. (1974). A historical-phenomenological study of bodily pain in Western man. *Bulletin of the History of Medicine, 48*(4), 540–570.

Dind, C. (1985). *From nursing to torture.* Paper presented at the Quadrennial International Nursing Congress, Tel Aviv, June 14–17.

Donald, I. (1976). At the receiving end. *Scottish Medical Journal, 21*, 49–57.

Donaldson, N. E. (1987). The phenomenological method: Qualitatively advancing nursing science. In S. R. Gortner (Ed.), *Nursing science methods: A reader* (pp. 89–92). San Francisco: University of California School of Nursing.

Donovan, M. (1982). Cancer pain: You can help! *Nursing Clinics of North America, 17*(4), 713–728.

Dreyfus, H. (1984). *Why current studies of human capacities can never be scientific* (Berkley Cognitive Science Report No. 11). Berkley: University of California.

Edwards, R. B. (1984). Pain and the ethics of pain management. *Social Science and Medicine, 18*(6), 515–523.

Engelhardt, H. T. Jr (1980). Ethical issues in pain management. In H. W. Kosterlitz & L. Y Terenius (Eds.), *Pain and society* (pp. 461–480). Weinheim: Verlag Chemie.

Euswas, P. (1991). *A grounded theory of caring in nursing practice.* Unpublished doctoral dissertation, Massey University, Palmerston North, New Zealand.

Fagerhaugh, S. Y., & Strauss, A. (1977). *Politics of pain management: Staff-patient interaction.* Menlo Park, CA: Addison-Wesley.

Farnsworth, K. E. (1985). Furthering the kingdom in psychology. In A. Holmes (Ed.), *The making of a Christian mind* (pp. 81–103). Downers Grove, IL: Inter Varsity Press.

Fields, H. L. (1987). *Pain.* New York: McGraw-Hill.

Fitzgerald, K. A. (1989). Burns. In B. Riegel & D. Ehrenreich (Eds.), *Psychological aspects of critical care nursing* (pp. 234–256). Rockville, MD: Aspen Publishers.

Forlini, J., Morin, D. M., & Treacy, S. (1987). Painless peds procedures. *American Journal of Nursing, 87*(3), 321–323.

Freed, D. L. J. (1975). Inadequate analgesia at night. *The Lancet, 1,* 519–520.

Gadow, S. (1980), Existential advocacy: Philosophical foundation of nursing. In S. F. Spiker & S. Gadow (Eds.), *Nursing, images and ideals* (pp. 79–101). New York: Springer.

Gadow, S. (1984). Touch and technology: Two paradigms of patient care. *Journal of Religion and Health, 23*(1), 63–69.

Gadow, S. (1986). Advocacy and paternalism in cancer nursing. In R. McCorkle & G. Hongladarom (Eds.), *Issues and topics in cancer nursing* (pp. 19–28). New York: Appleton-Century-Crofts.

Gadow, S. (1989). Clinical subjectivity: Advocacy with silent patients. *Nursing Clinics of North America, 24*(2), 535–541.

Gaines, A. D. (1985). The once- and the twice-born: Self and practice among psychiatrists and Christian psychiatrists. In R. A. Hahn & A. D. Gaines (Eds.), *Physicians of Western medicine: Anthropological approaches to theory and practice* (pp. 223–243). Dordrecht, Holland: D. Reidel Pub. Co.

Gottlieb, L., & Rowat, K. (1987). The McGill model of nursing: A practice-derived model. *Advances in Nursing Science, 9*(4), 51–61.

Guba, E. G., & Lincoln, Y. S. (1981). *Effective evaluation*. San Francisco: Jossey-Bass.

Haase, J. E. (1987). Components of courage in chronically ill adolescents: A phenomenological study. *Advances in Nursing Science, 9*(2), 64–80.

Hauck, S. L. (1986). Pain: Problem for the person with cancer. *Cancer Nursing, 9*(2), 66–76.

Heidegger, M. (1962). *Being and time*. New York: Harper & Row.

Heidrich, G., Perry, S., & Amand, R. (1981). Nursing staff attitudes about burn pain. *Journal of Burn Care and Rehabilitation, 2*(5), 259–261.

Hutchinson, M., & King, A. H. (1983). A nursing perspective on bone marrow transplantation. *Nursing Clinics of North America, 18*(3), 511–522.

Iafrati, N. S. (1986). Pain on the burn unit: Patient vs nurse perceptions. *Journal of Burn Care and Rehabilitation, 7*, 413–416.

International Association for the Study of Pain; Subcommittee on Taxonomy. (1979). Pain terms: A list with definitions and notes on usage. *Pain, 6*, 249–252.

Jay, S. M., Elliot, C., & Varni, J. W. (1986). Acute and chronic pain in adults and children with cancer. *Journal of Consulting and Clinical Psychology, 54*(5), 601–607.

Johnson, C. L., & Cain, V. J. (1985). CE Burn care: The rehab guide. *American Journal of Nursing, 85*(1), 48–50.

Jonsen, A. R. (1978). Do no harm. *Annals of Internal Medicine, 88,* 827–832.

Katz, E. R., Kellerman, J., & Siegel, S. E. (1980). Behavioral distress in children with cancer undergoing medical procedures: Developmental considerations. *Journal of Consulting and Clinical Psychology, 48*(3), 356–365.

Kelley, M. L., Jarvie, G. J., Middlebrook, J. L., McNeer, M. F., & Drabman, R. S. (1984). Decreasing burned children's pain behavior: Impacting the trauma of hydrotherapy. *Journal of Applied Behavior Analysis, 17*(2), 147–158.

Kesselring, A. (1990). *The experienced body, when taken-for-grantedness falters: A phenomenological study of living with breast cancer.* Unpublished doctoral dissertation, University of California, San Francisco.

Klein, R. M., & Charlton, J. E. (1980). Behavioral observation and analysis of pain behavior in critically burned patients. *Pain, 9,* 27–40.

Knafl, K. A., & Breitmayer, B. J. (1991). Triangulation in qualitative research: Issues of conceptual clarity and purpose. In J. M. Morse (Ed.), *Qualitative nursing research: A contemporary dialogue* (Rev. ed., pp. 226–239). Newbury Park, CA: Sage Publications.

Knafl, K. A., & Webster, D. C. (1988). Managing and analyzing data: A description of tasks, techniques, and materials. *Western Journal of Nursing Research, 10*(2), 195–218.

Krant, M. J. (1980). Oh, death—where is thy sting? In L. K. Y. Ng & J. J. Bonica (Eds.), *Pain, discomfort and humanitarian care* (pp. 313–328). New York: Elsevier North Holland.

Kwant, R. C. (1967). Merleau-Ponty and phenomenology. In J. J. Kockelmans (Ed.), *Phenomenology: The philosophy of Edmund Husserl and its interpretation* (pp. 375–392). Garden City, NY: Anchor Books.

Langer, M. M. (1989). *Merleau-Ponty's Phenomenology of perception: A guide and commentary*. London: Macmillan Press.

Lawler, J. (1997). *The body in nursing*. Melbourne: Churchill Livingstone.

Leder, D. (1984). Medicine and paradigms of embodiment. *Journal of Medicine and Philosophy, 9*(1), 29–43.

Leder, D. (1990). *The absent body*. Chicago: The University of Chicago Press.

Leininger, M. M. (1978). *Transcultural nursing: Concepts, theories, and practices*. New York: John Wiley & Sons.

Leonard, V. W. (1989). A Heideggerian phenomenologic perspective on the concept of the person. *Advances in Nursing Science, 11*(4), 40–55.

Lewis, C. S. (1962). *The problem of pain*. Glasgow: Fontana Books.

Lieb, I. C. (1976). The image of man in medicine. *Journal of Medicine and Philosophy, 1*(2), 162–176.

Lionberger, H. J. (1985). *An interpretive study of nurses practice of therapeutic touch*. Unpublished doctoral dissertation, University of California, San Francisco.

Lipton, S. (1987). Neurodestructive procedures in the management of cancer pain. *Journal of Pain and Symptom Management, 2*(4), 219–228.

Loeser, J. D., & Black, R. G. (1975). A taxonomy of pain. *Pain, 1*, 81–85.

Lowles, I. E., Al-Kurdi, M., & Hare, M. J. (1983). Women's recollection of pain during and after carbon dioxide laser treatment to the uterine cervix. *British Journal of Obstetrics and Gynaecology, 90*, 1157–1159.

Luckman, J., & Sorensen, K. (1980). *Medical-surgical nursing: The psychophysiological perspective*. Philadelphia: WB Saunders.

Lundin, R., Thiselton, A. C., & Walhout, C. (1985). *The responsibility of hermeneutics*. Grand Rapids, MI: WB Eerdmans Publ. Co.

Lynch-Sauer, J. (1985). Using a phenomenological research method to study nursing phenomena. In M. M. Leininger (Ed.), *Qualitative research methods in nursing* (pp. 93–107). New York: Grune & Stratton.

MacInnes, C. (1976). Cancer ward. *New Society, 29*(April), 232–234.

MacKinnon, B. (1988). On not harming: Two traditions. *The Journal of Medicine and Philosophy, 13*, 313–328.

Madjar, I. (1981). *The experience of pain in surgical patients: A cross-cultural comparison*. Unpublished master's thesis, Department of Nursing Studies, Massey University, Palmerston North, New Zealand.

Madjar, I. (1985). Pain and the surgical patient: A cross-cultural perspective. *The Australian Journal of Advanced Nursing, 2*(2), 29–33.

Madjar, I. (1987). Acute pain: Trivial or traumatic? *Nursing Praxis in New Zealand, 2*(3), 25–29.

Madjar, I. (1997). The body in health, illness and pain. In J. Lawler (Ed.), *The body in nursing* (pp. 53–73). Melbourne: Churchill Livingstone.

Marcel, G. (1960). *Mystery of being*. Chicago: Henry Regnery Co. (Gateway edition)

Marcel, G. (1965). *Being and having*. London: Collins. (Fontana edition)

Marcel, G. (1984a). Reply to J.B. O'Malley (Marcel's notion of a person). In P. A. Schilpp & L. E. Hahn (Eds.), *The philosophy of Gabriel Marcel* (p. 294). La Salle, IL: Open Court Publishing Co.

Marcel, G. (1984b). Reply to R.M. Zaner (The mystery of the body-qua-mine). In P. A. Schilpp & L. E. Hahn (Eds.), *The philosophy of Gabriel Marcel* (pp. 334–335). La Salle, IL: Open Court Publishing Co.

Marvin, J. A., & Heimbach, D. M. (1985). Pain control during the intensive care phase of burn care. *Critical Care Clinics, 1*(1), 147–157.

Massarik, F. (1981). The interviewing process re-visited. In P. Reason & J. Rowan (Eds.), *Human inquiry: A source book of new paradigm research* (pp. 201–206). New York: John Wiley & Sons.

Mather, L. E., & Mackie, J. (1983). The incidence of postoperative pain in children. *Pain, 15,* 271–282.

Mather, L. E., & Phillips, G. D. (1986). Opioids and adjuvants: Principles of use. In M. J. Cousins & G. D. Phillips (Eds.), *Acute pain management* (pp. 77–103). New York: Churchill Livingstone.

Mayer, D. K. (1986). Cancer patients' and families' perceptions of nurse caring behaviors. *Topics in Clinical Nursing, 8*(2), 63–69.

McConville, M. (1978). The phenomenological approach to perception. In R. S. Valle & M. King (Eds.), *Existential-phenomenological alternatives for psychology* (pp. 94–118). New York: Oxford University Press.

McGivney, W. T., & Crooks, G. M. (1984). The care of patients with severe chronic pain in terminal illness. *Journal of the American Medical Association, 251*(9), 1182–1188.

Melzack, R. (1973). *The puzzle of pain.* New York: Basic Books.

Melzack, R. (1975). The McGill pain questionnaire: Major properties and scoring methods. *Pain, 1,* 277–299.

Melzack, R. (1984). The myth of painless childbirth. *Pain, 19,* 331–337.

Melzack, R., & Wall, P. D. (1965). Pain mechanisms: A new theory. *Science, 150,* 971–979.

Melzack, R., & Wall, P. D. (1988). *The challenge of pain* (Rev. ed.). London: Penguin Books.

Menges, L. J. (1984). Pain, still an intriguing puzzle. *Social Science and Medicine, 19*(12), 1257–1260.

Merleau-Ponty, M. (1962). *Phenomenology of perception* (C. Smith, Trans.). New York: Routledge & Kegan Paul.

Merleau-Ponty, M. (1965). *The structure of behavior* (A. L. Fisher, Trans.). London: Methuen.

Merskey, H. (1980). The nature of pain. In W. L. Smith, H. Merskey, & S. C. Gross (Eds.), *Pain: Meaning and management* (pp. 71–74). New York: SP Medical and Scientific Books.

Merskey, H. (1982). Body-mind dilemma in chronic pain. In R. Roy & E. Tunks (Eds.), *Chronic pain: Psychological factors in rehabilitation* (pp. 10–19). Baltimore: Williams & Wilkins.

Merskey, H. (1984). Symptoms that depress the doctor: Too much pain. *British Journal of Hospital Medicine, 31*(1), 63–66.

Miles, M. B., & Huberman, A. M. (1984). *Qualitative data analysis: A source book of new methods.* Beverly Hills, CA: Sage Publications.

Miser, A. W., Dothage, J. A., Wesley, R. A., & Miser, J. S. (1987). The prevalence of pain in a pediatric and young adult cancer population. *Pain, 29,* 73–83.

Miser, A. W., McCalla, J., Dothage, J. A., Wesley, M., & Miser, J. S. (1987). Pain as a presenting symptom in children and young adults with newly diagnosed malignancy. *Pain, 29,* 85–90.

Morgan, J. P. (1986). American opiophobia: Customary underutilization of opioid analgesics. *Advances in Alcohol and Substance Abuse, 5*(1&2), 163–173.

Morse, J. M. (1989a). Qualitative nursing research: A free-for-all? In J. M. Morse (Ed.), *Qualitative nursing research: A contemporary dialogue* (pp. 3–10). Rockville, MD: Aspen Publishers.

Morse, J. M. (1989b). Strategies for sampling. In J. M. Morse (Ed.), *Qualitative nursing research: A contemporary dialogue* (pp. 117–131). Rockville, MD: Aspen Publishers.

Moss, D. (1978). Brain, body, and world: Perspectives on body-image. In R. S. Valle & M. King (Eds.), *Existential-phenomenological alternatives for psychology* (pp. 73–93). New York: Oxford University Press.

Munhall, P. L. (1989). Philosophical ponderings on qualitative research methods in nursing. *Nursing Science Quarterly, 2*(1), 20–28.

Munhall, P. L., & Oiler, C. J. (1986). Philosophical foundations of qualitative research. In P. L. Munhall & C. J. Oiler (Eds.), *Nursing research: A qualitative perspective* (pp. 47–63). Norwalk, CT: Appleton-Century-Crofts.

Murphy, G. J. (1989). Management of craniofacial pain with transcutaneous electrical nerve stimulation: A clinical protocol. *Journal of Pain and Symptom Management, 4*(1), 41–43.

Murphy, R. F. (1987). *The body silent.* New York: Henry Holt and Company.

New Zealand Nurses' Association. (1984). *Nursing education in New Zealand: A review and a statement of policy.* Wellington: Author.

Newman, M. A. (1986). *Health as expanding consciousness.* St Louis: C.V. Mosby Co.

Ng, L. K. Y. (1980). Pain and well-being: A challenge for biomedicine. In L. K. Y. Ng & J. J. Bonica (Eds.), *Pain, discomfort and humanitarian care* (pp. 353–365). New York: Elsevier North Holland.

Nightingale, F. (1970). *Notes on nursing: What it is and what it is not.* London: Duckworth.

Noordenbos, W. (1987). Some historical aspects. *Pain, 29,* 141–150.

Offsay, J. B. (1989). The pain of childhood leukemia: A parent's recollection. *Journal of Pain and Symptom Management, 4*(4), 174–178.

Oiler, C. J. (1986). Phenomenology: The method. In P. L. Munhall & C. J. Oiler. (Eds.), *Nursing research: A qualitative perspective* (pp. 69–84). Norwalk, CT: Appleton-Century-Crofts.

Omery, A. (1983). Phenomenology: A method for nursing research. *Advances in Nursing Science, 5*(2), 49–63.

Orem, D. E. (1985). *Nursing: Concepts of practice* (3rd ed.). New York: McGraw-Hill.

Orlando, I. J. (1961). *The dynamic nurse-patient relationship*. New York: Putnam's.

Orne, M. T., & Dinges, D. F. (1989). Hypnosis. In P. D. Wall & R. Melzack (Eds.), *Textbook of pain* (2nd ed., pp. 1021–1031). Edinburgh: Churchill Livingstone.

Over, R. (1980). Clinical and experimental pain. In C. Peck & M. Wallace (Eds.), *Problems in pain* (pp. 94–100). Sydney: Pergamon Press.

Parse, R. R. (1987). *Nursing science: Major paradigms, theories, and critiques*. Philadelphia: W.B. Saunders.

Peele, S. (1981). Reductionism in the psychology of the eighties: Can biochemistry eliminate addiction, mental illness, and pain? *American Psychologist, 36*(8), 807–818.

Perry, S. W. (1984a). Management of debridement pain. *PRN Forum, 3*(3), 1–3.

Perry, S. W. (1984b). Undermedication for pain on a burn unit. *General Hospital Psychiatry, 6*, 308–316.

Perry, S. W. (1984c). Frontiers in understanding burn injury. *The Journal of Trauma, 24*(Suppl. 9), S191–S195.

Perry, S. W., Cella, D. F., Falkenberg, J., Heidrich, G., & Goodwin, C. (1987). Pain perception in burn patients with stress disorder. *Journal of Pain and Symptom Management, 2*(1), 29–33.

Perry, S. W., & Heidrich, G. (1982). Management of pain during debridement: A survey of U.S. burn units. *Pain, 13*, 267–280.

Perry, S., Heidrich, G., & Ramos, E. (1981). Assessment of pain by burn patients. *Journal of Burn Care and Rehabilitation, 2*(6), 322–326.

Peteet, J., Tay, V., Cohen, G., & MacIntyre, J. (1986). Pain characteristics and treatment in an outpatient cancer population. *Cancer, 57*, 1259–1265.

Pinnick, N. J. (1984). *Coping behaviors of school-age children who undergo repeated intravenous procedures.* Unpublished master's thesis, University of California, San Francisco.

Polanyi, M. (1958). *Personal knowledge.* London: Routledge & Kegan Paul.

Prior, W. J. (1989). Compassion: A critique of moral rationalism. In R. L. Taylor & J. Watson (Eds.), *They shall not hurt: Human suffering and human caring* (pp. 33–51). Boulder, CO: Colorado Associated University Press.

Procacci, P. (1980). History of the pain concept. In H. W. Kosterlitz & L. Y. Terenius (Eds.), *Pain and society* (pp. 3–12). Weinheim: Verlag Chemie.

Procacci, P., & Maresca, M. (1984). Pain concept in Western civilization: A historical review. In C. Benedetti, C. R. Chapman, & G. Moricca (Eds.), *Advances in pain research and therapy* (Vol. 7, pp. 1–11). New York: Raven Press.

Ray, M. A. (1985). A philosophical method to study nursing phenomena. In M. M. Leininger (Ed.), *Qualitative research methods in nursing* (pp. 81–91). New York: Grune & Stratton.

Reinharz, S. (1983). Phenomenology as a dynamic process. *Phenomenology + Pedagogy, 1*(1), 77–79.

Riemen, D. J. (1986a). The essential structure of a caring interaction: Doing phenomenology. In P. L. Munhall & C. J. Oiler (Eds.), *Nursing research: A qualitative perspective* (pp. 85–108). Norwalk, CT: Appleton-Century-Crofts.

Riemen, D. J. (1986b). Noncaring and caring in the clinical setting: Patients' descriptions. *Topics in Clinical Nursing, 8*(2), 30–36.

Robertson, K. E., Cross, P. J., & Terry, J. C. (1985). CE Burn care: The crucial first days. *American Journal of Nursing, 85*(1), 29–47.

Roy, C. (1976). *Introduction to nursing: An adaptation model.* Englewood Cliffs, NJ: Prentice-Hall.

Ryle, G. (1976). Phenomenology. In H. D. Durfee (Ed.), *Analytic philosophy and phenomenology* (pp. 17–28). The Hague: Martinus Nijhoff.

Sacks, O. (1984). *A leg to stand on.* London: Pan Books. (Picador edition)

Salsberry, P. J. (1989). Phenomenological research in nursing: Commentary: Fundamental issues. *Nursing Science Quarterly, 2*(1), 9–13.

Sandelowski, M. (1986). The problem of rigor in qualitative research. *Advances in Nursing Science, 8*(3), 27–37.

Sandelowski, M., & Pollock, C. (1986). Women's experiences of infertility. *Image, 18*(4), 140–144.

Scarry, E. (1985). *The body in pain.* New York: Oxford University Press.

Schreml, W. (1984). Pain in the cancer patient as a consequence of therapy (surgery, radiotherapy, chemotherapy). *Recent Results in Cancer Research, 89,* 85–99.

Siddle, N. C., Young, O., Sledmere, C. M., Reading, A. E., & Whitehead, M. I. (1983). A controlled trial of naproxen sodium for relief of pain associated with Vabra suction curettage. *British Journal of Obstetrics and Gynaecology, 90,* 864–869.

Skrzynecki, P. (1987). *The wild dogs.* St Lucia, Qld: University of Queensland Press.

Smith, J. K., & Heshusius, L. (1986). Closing down the conversation: The end of the quantitative-qualitative debate among educational inquirers. *Educational Researcher, 15,* 4–12.

Smith, M. C. (1989). Phenomenological research in nursing: Response: Facts about phenomenology in nursing. *Nursing Science Quarterly, 2*(1), 13–16.

Solem, L. D. (1987). Thermal injuries. In F. B. Cerra (Ed.), *Manual of critical care* (pp. 585–593). St Louis: C.V. Mosby & Co.

Spiegelberg, H. (1969). *The phenomenological movement: A historical introduction* (2nd ed.). The Hague: Martinus Nijhoff.

Spiro, H. M. (1976). Pain and perfectionism—The physician and the "pain patient." *The New England Journal of Medicine, 294*(15), 829–830.

Sriwatanakul, K., Weis, O. F., Alloza, J. L., Kelvie, W., Weintraub, M., & Lasagna, L. (1983). Analysis of narcotic analgesic usage in the treatment of postoperative pain. *Journal of the American Medical Association, 250*(7), 926–929.

Stainton, M. C. (1985). *Origins of attachment: Culture and cue sensitivity.* Unpublished doctoral dissertation, University of California, San Francisco.

Stern, P. N. (1991). Are counting and coding a cappela appropriate in qualitative research. In J. M. Morse (Ed.), *Qualitative nursing research: A contemporary dialogue* (Rev. ed., pp. 147–162). Newbury Park, CA: Sage Publications.

Sternbach, R. A. (1974). *Pain patients: Traits and treatment.* New York: Academic Press.

Stewart, D., & Mickunas, A. (1974). *Exploring phenomenology: A guide to the field and its literature.* Chicago: American Library Association.

Straus, E. W. (1966). *Phenomenological psychology.* London: Tavistock Publications.

Straus, E. W., & Machado, M. A. (1984). Gabriel Marcel's notion of incarnate being. In P. A. Schilpp & L. E. Hahn (Eds.), *The philosophy of Gabriel Marcel* (pp. 123–155). La Salle, IL: Open Court Publishing Co.

Styles, M. M. (1982). *On nursing: Toward a new endowment.* St Louis: CV Mosby.

Swanson, J. M., & Chenitz, W. C. (1982). Why qualitative research in nursing? *Nursing Outlook, 30*(4), 241–245.

Swanson-Kauffman, K., & Schonwald, E. (1988). Phenomenology. In B. Sarter (Ed.), *Paths to knowledge: Innovative research methods for nursing* (pp. 97–105). New York: National League for Nursing.

Tagore, R. (1916/1985). *The home and the world.* Harmondsworth, England: Penguin Books.

Taylor, A. G., Skelton, J. A., & Butcher, J. (1984). Duration of pain condition and physical pathology as determinants of nurses' assessments of patients in pain. *Nursing Research, 33*(1), 4–8.

Teske, K., Daut, R. L., & Cleeland, C. S. (1983). Relationships between nurses' observations and patients' self-reports of pain. *Pain, 16,* 289–296.

Tisdale, S., (1986). *The sorcerer's apprentice: Tales of the modern hospital.* New York: McGraw-Hill.

Tobiasen, J. M., & Hiebert, J. M. (1985). Burns and adjustment to injury: Do psychological strategies help? *The Journal of Trauma, 25*(12), 1151–1155.

Tolstoy, L. (1918/1973). *Anna Karenina.* London: Oxford University Press.

Toombs, S. K. (1987). The meaning of illness: A phenomenological approach to the patient-physician relationship. *The Journal of Medicine and Philosophy, 12,* 219–240.

Travelbee, J. (1971). *Interpersonal aspects of nursing* (2nd ed.). Philadelphia: F.A. Davis.

Tu, W. (1980). A religiophilosophical perspective on pain. In H. W. Kosterlitz & L. Y. Terenius (Eds.), *Pain and society* (pp. 63–78). Weinheim: Verlag Chemie.

Turk, D. C., & Kerns, R. D. (1984). Conceptual issues in the assessment of clinical pain. *International Journal of Psychiatry in Medicine, 13*(1), 57–68.

Van der Does, A. J. W. (1989). Patients' and nurses' ratings of pain and anxiety during burn wound care. *Pain, 39,* 95–101.

van Manen, M. (1984). *"Doing" phenomenological research and writing: An introduction* (Monograph No. 7). Edmonton: Department of Secondary Education, University of Alberta.

van Manen, M. (1990). *Researching lived experience.* London, Ontario: The Althouse Press.

Wakeman, R. J., & Kaplan, J. Z. (1978). An experimental study of hypnosis in painful burns. *American Journal of Clinical Hypnosis, 21*(1), 3–12.

Waldman, S. D., Feldstein, G. S., & Allen, M. L. (1987). Neuroadenolysis of the pituitary: Description of a modified technique. *Journal of Pain and Symptom Management, 2*(1), 45–49.

Walkenstein, M. D. (1982). Comparison of burned patients' perception of pain with nurses' perception of patients' pain. *Journal of Burn Care and Rehabilitation, 3*(4), 233–236.

Wall, P. D. (1984). Neurophysiology of acute and chronic pain. In C. Benedetti, C. R. Chapman, & G. Moricca (Eds.), *Advances in pain research and therapy* (Vol. 7, pp. 13–25). New York: Raven Press.

Wild, J. (1965). Foreword. In M. Merleau-Ponty (Ed.), *The structure of behavior* (A. L. Fisher, Trans., pp. xii–xvii). London: Methuen.

Williams, R. S. (1984). Ability, disability and rehabilitation: A phenomenological description. *Journal of Medicine and Philosophy, 9*(1), 93–112.

Welch-McCaffrey, D. (1986). Role performance issues for oncology clinical nurse specialists. *Cancer Nursing, 9*(6), 287–294.

White, M. (1972). Importance of selected nursing activities. *Nursing Research, 21*, 4–14.

Wolf, Z. R. (1986). The caring concept and nurse identified caring behaviors. *Topics in Clinical Nursing, 8*(2), 84–93.

Wooldridge-King, M. (1982). Nursing considerations of the burned patient during the emergent period. *Heart & Lung, 11*(4), 353–363.

Wuthnow, R., Hunter, J. D., Bergesen, A., & Kurzweil, E. (1984). *Cultural analysis: The work of Peter L. Berger, Mary Douglas, Michel Foucault, and Jurgen Habermas.* London: Routledge & Kegan Paul.

Zaner, R. M. (1964). *The problem of embodiment.* The Hague: Martinus Nijhoff.

Index